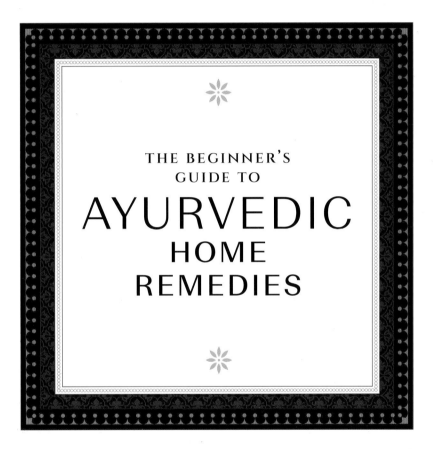

THE BEGINNER'S
GUIDE TO

AYURVEDIC
HOME
REMEDIES

To Larry, for making our home a healing place and our hearts a loving space.

Quarto.com

© 2023 Quarto Publishing Group USA Inc.
Text © 2023 Susan Weis-Bohlen

First Published in 2023 by Fair Winds Press, an imprint of The Quarto Group,
100 Cummings Center, Suite 265-D, Beverly, MA 01915, USA.
T (978) 282-9590 F (978) 283-2742

Fair Winds Press titles are also available at discount for retail, wholesale, promotional, and bulk purchase. For details, contact the Special Sales Manager by email at specialsales@quarto.com or by mail at The Quarto Group, Attn: Special Sales Manager, 100 Cummings Center, Suite 265-D, Beverly, MA 01915, USA.

27 26 25 24 23   1 2 3 4 5

ISBN: 978-0-7603-8205-9

Digital edition published in 2023
eISBN: 978-0-7603-8206-6

Library of Congress Cataloging-in-Publication Data is available.

Cover Design: Landers Miller Design
Page Layout: Megan Jones Design
Photography: Shutterstock. Getty Images pages 16 and 44. Background on pages 4–5 by Hendrik Kespohl on Unsplash.
Illustration: Maggie Cote

Printed in China

The information in this book is for educational purposes only and is not intended to replace the advice of a physician or medical practitioner. Do not attempt to treat serious injuries or illnesses with Ayurveda alone. Be aware that Ayurveda is not a licensed profession in the US. When visiting a practitioner, ask for their certifications and affiliations to national associations to help you decide if they are right for you. Additionally, training for yoga teachers varies widely. A teacher with at least 500 hours of training is preferable. All case studies and descriptions of persons have been changed or altered to be unrecognizable. Any likeness to actual persons, living or dead, is strictly coincidental.

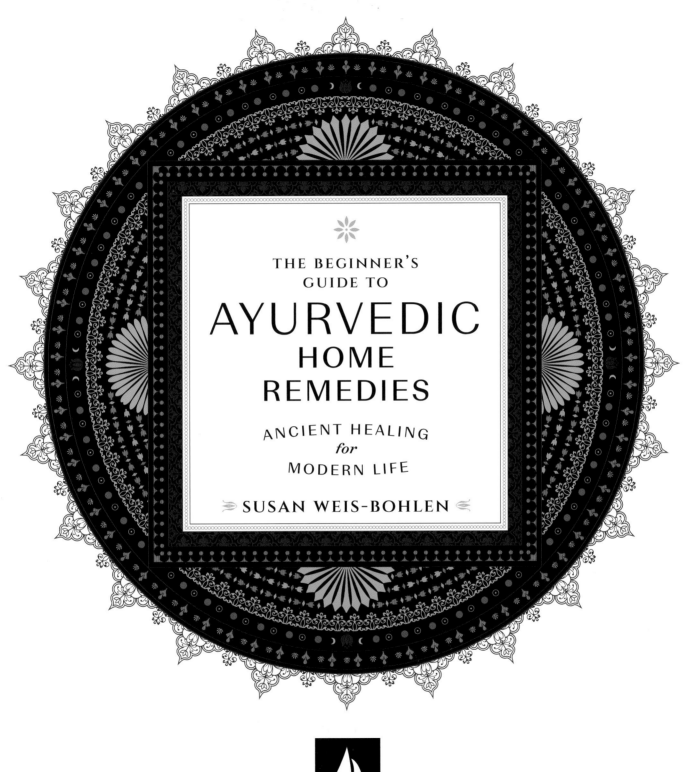

THE BEGINNER'S
GUIDE TO

AYURVEDIC
HOME
REMEDIES

ANCIENT HEALING
for
MODERN LIFE

⇒ SUSAN WEIS-BOHLEN ⇐

FAIR WINDS

Contents

Introduction:
Ayurveda: Ancient Science
in Modern Times

7

Chapter 1

Sleep:
Optimal Rest and Restoration

17

Chapter 2

Pain:
Mind and Body Relief

45

Chapter 3

Respiratory System:
Breathing into Perfect Health

65

Chapter 4

Digestion:
Mouth, Gut, Assimilation,
and Elimination

87

Chapter 5

....

Skin:
The Body's Largest Organ

123

Chapter 6

....

Reproductive System:
Healthy for Life

147

Chapter 7

....

**Caring for Yourself and Others
at Every Age**

171

Resources   **184**

Acknowledgments   **186**

About the Author   **187**

Index   **188**

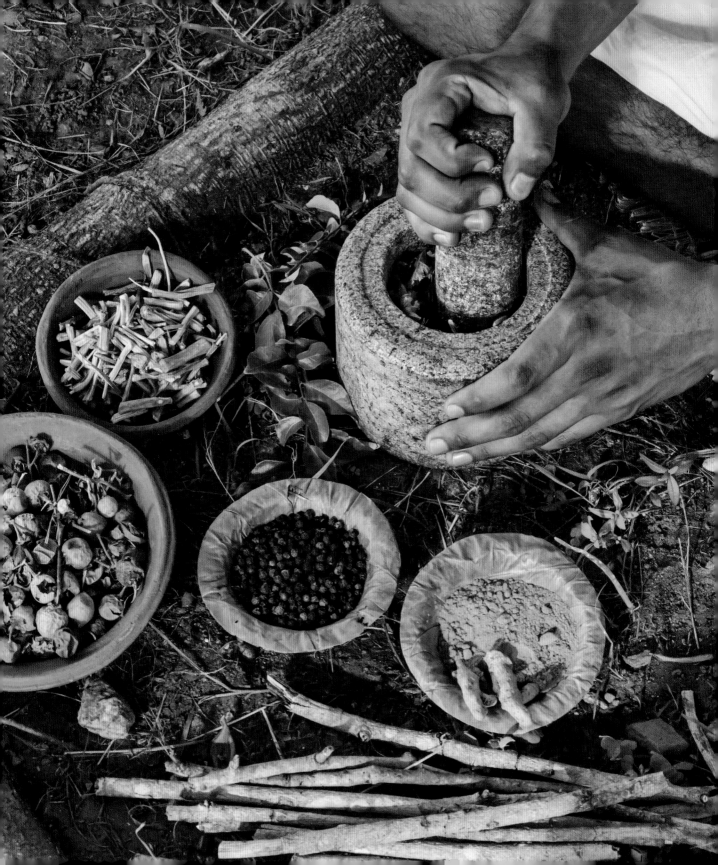

Introduction

Ayurveda: Ancient Science in Modern Times

Ayurveda has existed for more than 5,000 years. Often called the science of life, it has its roots in India, and it has been used around the world to cultivate healing and balance. In 2007, I began exploring this incredible practice of health, longevity, and living in harmony with nature. I was drawn to the promise of self-care, sustainable practices, and disease prevention that Ayurveda offered.

At the time, I was a forty-four-year-old bookstore owner, working six or seven days a week, sometimes more than twelve hours a day. I lived alone and ran my shop mostly on my own, with the help of a few part-timers. Owning the bookstore was a dream and was truly fulfilling, but I was stressed, drained, and weary. I had about fifty extra pounds on my body, and on my way home late at night I would be starved and exhausted and, once in a while, I would even stop at a fast-food drive-thru to get fries or a shake.

My store was a new-age bookshop that had books on everything from angels and aromatherapy to meditation, yoga, and vegetarian cooking—and even a small section on Ayurveda. I had been meditating and doing yoga for more than twenty years, and I had heard Ayurveda called a sister science to those modalities. Drawn to learn more, I borrowed a few books from the shop, and I took a *dosha* quiz to learn my unique combination of elements.

Dosha is Sanskrit for mind/body constitution. My dosha illuminated why I held on to weight, had trouble saying no, took care of others before myself, and sometimes felt intense anger, frustration, and impatience. I had many traits that indicated my *Kapha/Pitta* energies were out of balance.

I was tired of being overweight, and I knew deep down that the girl who excelled at yoga and swimming, and who loved to be outdoors, could do all those things more comfortably with less weight on her body. In my early thirties, I weighed as much as 237 pounds (108 kg). Even at 5'7" (170 cm), that felt like it was too much for me, but every time I tried to lose weight, I became bulimic. The pressure to keep the weight off, especially using brand-name diet plans, left me feeling deprived and starved.

Rather than struggle with my weight, I instead entered into Ayurveda focused on detoxing—removing the blockages in my mind and body that left me feeling dissatisfied and unfulfilled. I felt like I had a sticky residue inside me that was keeping me from absorbing nutrients, experiences, and emotions. I wanted to clear the channels and fully embrace all life had to offer.

Healing the Imbalance

I can do this, I thought! As I entered this next stage in life, I wanted to be a reflection of how I knew I would feel if only I cleaned myself up inside and out. But I needed a little help to get started. For me, that meant having the detox treatment called *Panchakarma* (known as PK) at The Chopra Center Spa in San Diego, California. I hopped on a plane from Baltimore and began the journey of a lifetime.

The theory behind PK is five basic treatments to push toxins out of the mind and body while the patient rests and allows their system to repair, restore, and rejuvenate. Through oil massages, herbal enemas, and other treatments, I saw forty-four years of toxins leave my body—boxes of cookies, cartons of ice cream, and several bad relationships. As what no longer served me was expelled, I saw what could take its place: joy, healthy relationships, and nutritious food that fed my bones, blood, and tissues. PK made space for that to happen, pure and simple.

As I embraced Ayurveda, especially by eating for my dosha (Kapha-reducing) and practicing *abhyanga* (daily self-massage with oils), I felt satiated and nourished. I never felt deprived. I was more attuned to the needs, wants, and beauty of my body. There is nothing like massaging every nook and cranny daily, with oil, to really get to know and, hopefully, love yourself!

The weight came off as my body let go of toxins, almost as if it was the "symptom" rather than the "cause." The weight seemed to be the container of that sticky residue. By letting that go, my body came into balance, my mind became clear and focused, and my heart opened wide for whatever was coming next.

I lost those fifty extra pounds, and I emptied the cabinets of junk food. I bought mung beans, masoor dal lentils, and basmati rice. Ginger and turmeric roots, cumin, cardamom, and fennel seeds all found their way to my kitchen. I bought a pressure cooker, an immersion blender, and an Indian spice box. I learned how to prepare Ayurvedic meals from the experts and studied and received certifications in the United States and India and became an Ayurveda health counselor, a pulse and tongue reader, a Marma therapist, a cooking instructor, a teacher, a public speaker, and an author. And along the way I met the man I was going to marry at forty-five, and I got married at forty-seven.

Suddenly, Ayurveda no longer was something that repaired my health—it was a calling. I felt enlisted to bring my voice and experiences to the practice and share what I learned with the world. I know that not everyone can take off twenty-one days to get PK, and not everyone has an Ayurvedic practitioner in their town. My intention, then and now, is to ease you into this ancient practice of a consciousness-based spiritual and medical science. With the information and resources presented here, I hope that you'll be motivated, excited, and encouraged, as you see the possibilities for healing yourself, your family, and even your community.

Food, Lifestyle, and Apothecary

This book is designed to help you find your way into the practice, to see how a three-tiered plan of food, lifestyle, and apothecary can create balance and harmony in mind, body, and spirit. It will show you how simple adjustments can heal common conditions and ailments and how you can do this on your own.

Many of us have had the experience of Western, allopathic medicine falling short, leaving us without a diagnosis or a clear plan to follow. Often, it is only the symptom that is treated, not the underlying cause. For example, you suddenly have painful hives around your belly and upper thighs, so you visit a dermatologist. The result might be a prescription for a steroid cream, and you'll be out of there in fifteen minutes, max. But what about the food you eat, the detergent you use, or your stress levels? When did the hives appear, and has this happened before? A functional medicine doctor, a naturopath, a Chinese medicine practitioner, or an Ayurvedic practitioner would understand the hives to be a symptom of something else going wrong in the mind or body, and they would work with you to treat the root cause.

What Is Ayurveda?

Ayurveda is based on the five elements: space, air, fire, water, and earth. These building blocks of nature are the building blocks of life. Space and air offer us freedom of movement, unlimited potential, and creativity. Fire ignites our minds, sparks digestion and metabolism, and creates light. Water and earth establish a cohesive structure, a foundation to build on, and a layer of protection.

We call these elemental combinations the doshas—Vata, Pitta, and Kapha—and we all have our own distinct composition of them. When we are balanced in our unique makeup, we feel strong in mind and body. When there is too much of a dosha, it may show up physically and/or mentally as illness, disease, or discomfort.

For example, you may be a thin, lanky person who forgets to eat and drink because your mind is always busy jumping from one idea or project to the next, leaving you excited about your creativity but ultimately depleted, lacking the energy to focus or complete a task, let alone feed and care for yourself. This is an example of too much Vata dosha—cold air and dry wind coursing through mind and body, disturbing the balance. This leads to disorders such as constipation, insomnia, and arthritis.

Dosha Quiz

Try this quiz here to begin the journey. Answer A, B, or C for how you have been for most of your life. This is called your *Prakruti*, your primary state of balance. Prakruti is how you have been for most of your life, your natural-born dosha. Take the quiz a second time, focusing on how you are currently feeling, which is called your *Vikruti*, or your natural-born mind/body constitution. Vikruti is your current state of being, and it will highlight where some imbalances may be in your life right now.

BODY TYPE

A) Lean and lanky
B) Strong, medium build
C) Heavy, full, large boned

WEIGHT

A) Low; hard to gain weight and keep it on
B) Normal for my height; stable
C) Heavy for my height; easy to gain, hard to lose

EYES

A) Squinty, small; wander when talking or listening
B) Sharp, intense; stare at people when talking or listening
C) Large, round; warm gaze

SLEEP

A) Difficult to fall asleep or stay asleep; mind races
B) Sleeps 5 to 6 hours a night; feels refreshed
C) Sleeps soundly for 9 or 10 hours; difficult to wake up

SKIN

A) Thin and cold to the touch; always needs an extra layer
B) Reddish; warm, even in cold weather
C) Thick, cool; clammy, slightly moist

BOWEL MOVEMENTS

A) Constipated; dry, hard stool; once a day or fewer
B) Loose and sometimes watery; several times a day
C) Well formed, large; once or twice a day

APPETITE

A) Sometimes feels hungry but forgets to eat
B) Wakes up ravenous and gets angry when hungry
C) Rarely hungry, but eats when the clock says to or food is present

UNDER STRESS

A) Scared, anxious, worried, confused
B) Angry, blames others, easily frustrated, impatient with self and others
C) Withdraws, blames self, eats to soothe

RESULTS

Total As: _____

Total Bs: _____

Total Cs: _____

If you have more As, you are primarily Vata.

More Bs, you are Pitta.

More Cs, you are Kapha.

Make a note of both your Prakruti and your Vikruti. It will come in handy as you read through the remedies and recommendations.

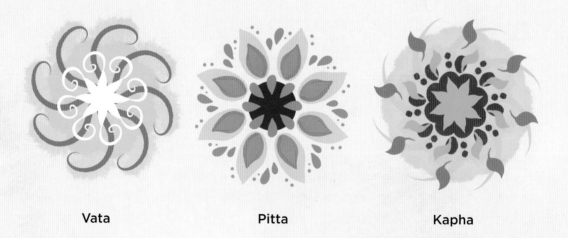

Vata   Pitta   Kapha

Or perhaps you are an athlete, perfectionist, or type A personality. The fire in your belly roars and is fed by intense activities, fierce competition, and winning. This potentially leads to excess fire presenting as anger, frustration, blame, and impatience with yourself or others when things don't go your way. This heat is excessive Pitta dosha. It may drive people away from you and cause migraines, skin rashes, hair loss, and digestive issues.

And then there is the nurturer, the caretaker, the one who, on an airplane, forgets to put their oxygen mask on first and insists on taking care of everyone else before taking care of themselves. The one who just doesn't say no, gets overwhelmed, and retreats and eats. Eventually, they become so stagnant that they no longer find the energy to help anyone or themselves. This is Kapha. Saturated in earth and water, they get heavy, lazy, and stuck and the skin is cool and clammy. The sinuses fill with mucus, a wet cough settles in, and seasonal allergies come around every year.

By doing the opposite—warmth and moisture for Vata, cooling and sweetness for Pitta, and dryness and warmth for Kapha—we heal. Determining your primary dosha helps you find your sweet spot where your unique elemental makeup is balanced. In this state of being, you are functioning at your optimal level, feeling rested and energized. Food is digested easily, you rarely get sick, and when you do, you recover more quickly.

Koshas and Dhatus

Ayurveda sees the human mind and body as a series of layers, or sheaths, we call *koshas*. The *anamaya kosha* is our skin; it is the layer derived from food. Next is the *pranayama kosha*. Prana means breath or life force. This is our energy layer. The *manomaya kosha* is the mind, intellect, and ego. Then we have the *vijnanamaya kosha*, which is where wisdom, discrimination, and intuition lie. The *anandamaya* is the bliss body, where our inner work aligns with the spiritual world.

We are both protected by and limited by our koshas. For example, when tightly bound in the manomaya kosha, we cling to our ideas and mindsets, and we shun others who don't share the same belief system. We limit our world to only those who think like we do. If we believe the ego defines our self-image by our possessions, the people we know, and our place in society, when those things are gone, we have nothing and are shattered.

Each kosha has a purpose, and if we live a life of generosity, curiosity, and compassion, we overcome the restraints of the koshas. How do we do that? Nearly every remedy and recommendation in this book aligns with breaking free from the limiting qualities of the koshas. We must eat, breathe, move, sleep, love, receive, and give mindfully, yielding when needed, responding to ourselves and others with a softness, a quality of understanding. When we do this, we nourish ourselves and others deeply. By dropping the ego and the sense of right and wrong, we see that most things in moderation are useful, and many things are both medicine and poison. Using antibiotics for a serious infection is medicine; using antibiotics for acne for twenty years is poison.

In addition to the sheaths of the kosha, Ayurveda identifies seven layers of tissue in the body, called the *dhatus* in Sanskrit. They are plasma, blood, muscle, fat, bone, marrow, and reproductive tissues. When absorption of nutrients and the ability to rid the body of toxins work well, the dhatus are nourished and balanced. The food we eat is assimilated, and the waste is readied for elimination through urine, feces, blood, and sweat. Simply, the food we eat must nourish all seven dhatus.

As ailments, issues, and conditions arise, take action immediately—before the problem settles deeply into the tissues. The longer we have the ailment, the deeper it digs and the more difficult it becomes to treat. At the first sign of a problem, notice it, address it. Don't hesitate. Reach out so that it does not fester, take root, and become more difficult to eradicate. What dosha seems to be out of balance? Are you able to figure out the cause and mitigate it? Or do you need help from a professional?

So we have koshas, dhatus, and the Ayurvedic pillars in life: diet, sleep, and sexual activity. When we have balance in these three areas, we are healthy, productive beings. Although sexual activity here means that we are able to procreate, I want to take it a step further and call it social activity. We must be a part of the world, engaged and useful, to fully be balanced. Sharing our lives in community, with a loved one, friends, family, pets, neighbors, or just recognizing the people we interact with but don't know well, this all fulfills our sense of belonging, which is necessary to be healthy and happy.

How to Use This Book

This book may be used as a prevention workbook and a manual for healthy living. You will find methods to boost your immunity and prevent disease by following proper guidelines for sleeping, eating, and exercising. I also share meditation practices and the application of oils to relieve pain, increase mobility, and soothe aches and pains. By incorporating these practices into your everyday life, you will get sick less often, heal faster, and feel deeply nourished. You also can use this book as a reference guide: Simply look up a condition, illness, or symptoms that are ailing you, and discover the remedies to help you as you need them.

Please be aware that this book is a beginner's guide to help you find relief from common ailments. If you are experiencing serious physical or mental illness, please contact a doctor or go to an emergency room. This book is not a substitute for acute care for life-threatening issues. An Ayurvedic practitioner may work with your doctor to support you, but currently Ayurveda is not a licensed practice in the United States. If you decide to work with an Ayurvedic practitioner, ask to see their certifications and research their school or program. Ask if they are a member of NAMA—the National Ayurvedic Medical Association. Knowing who your practitioner is will create trust and a bond as you work together toward perfect health.

Ayurveda says food is medicine, and we will talk a lot about food in this book. Try to buy or grow all organic food if possible. Look for non-genetically modified organisms and organic and local products. When shopping in the farmers' market, ask the vendors if their produce is organic. Use of glyphosate (like Roundup) and other chemicals is widely known to cause cancer, and it depletes the soil of nutrients. Remember that just because a product is non-GMO, it does not mean it is organic. The resources section (page 184) lists products I use myself and have been suggesting to my clients for years.

Look up something that has been irritating you. Learn how to bolster your immune system and create a healthier lifestyle. Take on just one or two ideas and see how it goes. It's surprising how quickly some Ayurvedic remedies take effect. Others may take a while to notice. After all, it may have taken years for certain ailments to manifest, so it might take a little while to ease the condition. Be patient. Stay the course. You'll most certainly reap the benefits and rewards of an Ayurvedic lifestyle for the rest of your life.

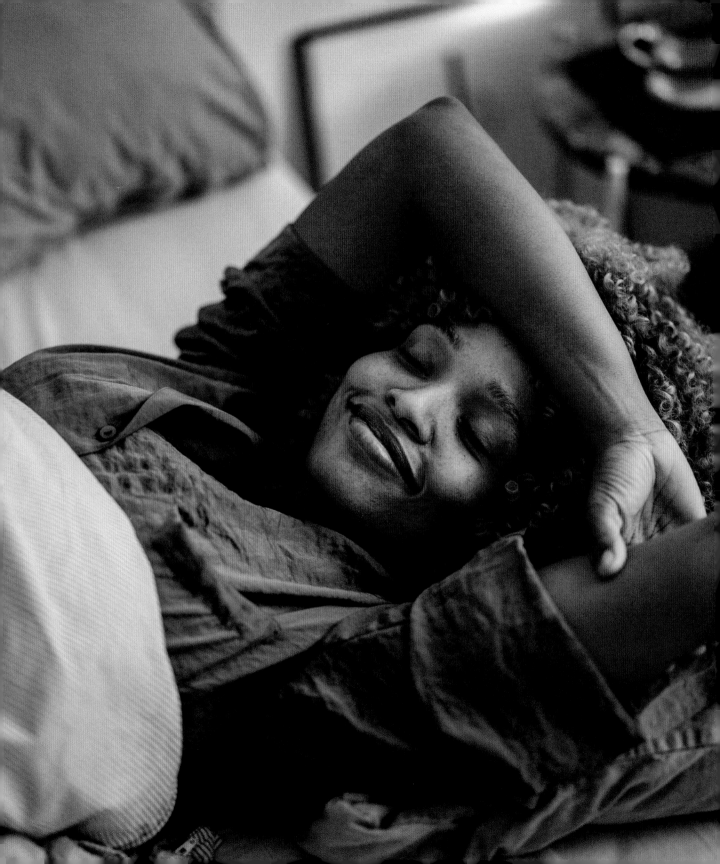

1

Sleep: Optimal Rest and Restoration

There is a sweet spot when it comes to sleep. Too much or too little will negatively affect your health. The food you eat, the time you eat it, when you go to sleep, and where you sleep all affect the quality of your rest. We'll explore sleep hygiene so that you can set yourself up for the most restorative rest. Then we'll address insomnia, sleep apnea, and nightmares, along with some Ayurvedic remedies to help you get back to restorative, peaceful sleep.

What Happens When We Sleep?

Good sleep helps ensure a robust immune system, an alert and focused mind, and great digestion. Yes, sleep even affects digestion, detoxification, and absorption of nutrients. There are four stages of sleep, and different functions occur in the mind and body at each stage.

- Waking consciousness: This is when we are awake, active, and aware of our surroundings.

- REM, or rapid eye movement: After we fall asleep, we may wake up to turn over, adjust the sheets, move the dog, or get up to pee. When we fall back to sleep, we enter the REM stage: This is where we dream, and the body is deeply relaxed. Your breath rate may accelerate and your eyes will flutter as you witness your dreams—even if you don't remember them.

- Light sleep: During this stage, when we are just falling asleep or back to sleep, we drift in and out and are awoken easily by sounds, lights, or movement.

- Deep sleep, or slow-wave sleep: We need time for the body to rest and digest, and deep sleep provides a restorative phase. The breath, heart rate, and pulse slow down. The brain is quiet, and the metabolic functions move toward completion, with waste being readied for elimination and nutrients assimilated into the tissues.

The time we spend in each stage depends on age, lifestyle, food, exercise, and overall state of health and well-being. From infancy to our teens, we need more sleep to promote proper physical and mental growth. As we get older, we tend to be more on the go with life, work, and other obligations, and we may sleep less, sometimes looking at sleep as a waste of time as there always seems like there is so much to do! That sleep deprivation comes with a cost that may show up in nearly every aspect of our health. In the later stages of life, deep sleep seems elusive, and even though we have more time and desire to rest, we might spend more time awake in bed than asleep.

Measure Your Stages of Sleep

There are several products on the market that can help you get a good sense of the quality of your sleep. A smart watch will monitor your sleep and give you a report in the morning. There are rings and bracelets that will track your sleep (as well as your steps, movements, and more). The reports are detailed, including heart rate, pulse, body temperature, blood oxygen levels, and more. Some will monitor heart rate variability (HRV): High HRV means you are responding and recovering well in various situations. A low HRV indicates you are in stress or recovery mode.

Learning your personal metrics may help you spot deficiencies and note where you are doing well. Some companies that make the sleep-measuring products offer support systems to help you make better choices. (The website thesleepdoctor.com has invaluable advice.)

Along with the phases of the moon and the ocean tides, the human body follows the rhythm of nature. Nature offers us a road map with circadian rhythms, the natural sleep-wake cycle that is part of the body's internal clock. Melatonin is a brain chemical that increases as the day darkens into night. The less light that enters the eyes, the more melatonin is produced, and the sleepier we get. We inhibit this reaction if we keep the lights burning and electronic screens on. It is so important to minimize these as we move into the evening because, with a little effort, we can help our bodies get back on track. Lower the lights, switch tablets and phones to night mode, and wind down naturally to increase melatonin in the brain.

There are basic guidelines to ensure a good night's sleep. By following the good sleep hygiene practices on page 21, you should be able to regulate your sleep at any age—knowing that as we age, our needs are different. A sixty-year-old will probably not sleep like a six- or sixteen-year-old! Follow the specific food, lifestyle, and supplement suggestions along with keeping up good sleep hygiene practices to ensure deep, healing rest.

THE VALUE OF DEEP SLEEP

Once you become familiar with your sleep patterns, whether by using a device or paying close attention to your waking/sleeping schedule, dig even deeper and see where you can make improvements. For example, many older people naturally get less "deep sleep" than younger people, but the deep sleep stage is highly restorative for brain cognition and repair of the tissues. It is being studied as a way to prevent Alzheimer's disease. In this stage, new memories are consolidated and processed. Failure to process these memories might lead to forgetfulness and impairments in memory categorization.

If you don't get enough deep sleep, try these methods:

- Focus on getting to bed a little earlier. This will give you more time to sink into deeper sleep. "Early to bed" is your mantra.

- Heat the body in the hours before bed by taking a warm bath, using a hot tub, or taking a sauna.

- Try quick, intense aerobic movements, such as jogging in place or using a rowing machine—just enough to feel the heat, maybe for 10 minutes, before bed. It's not exactly clear why heating the body works: When the body is hot, it tries to cool down, and we sleep better in a cooler environment, so this may be a factor. Note: If you have insomnia, exercise earlier in the day, as that intensity could keep you up at night.

Good Sleep Hygiene Practices

Because sleep is restorative for the mind and body, it is imperative that we spend a prescribed amount of time in each stage, every night, to receive maximum benefits. We simply cannot skimp on sleep and expect to be healthy. These strategies will help you obtain the best sleep.

FOOD: EATING FOR SLEEP

Eat your last meal at least 3 hours before bed. Going to bed on an empty stomach, for most people, makes it easier to fall asleep. If you are truly hungry before bed, have a handful of seeds or nuts, preferably unsalted, or a small bowl of popcorn or rice with a pat of ghee, olive oil, or butter.

Keep dinner/supper light and easy to digest. Choose light proteins such as fish, turkey, chicken, mung beans, or lentils. Eat steamed, roasted, or cooked veggies, with some complex carbohydrates. Avoid raw foods such as salad; raw food is harder to digest and will disrupt sleep. Leave out sugary, creamy desserts. Avoid wine and spirits. To further aid digestion, take a 5- to 10-minute easy-paced walk after eating.

Eat a wide variety of foods containing omegas. Omegas help the gut microbiome stay vibrant. Note: Omega-3s and omega-9s (fatty acids) help the body by reducing inflammation, regulating insulin, increasing memory, supporting mental health, and balancing sleep patterns. But not all omegas are equal. Omega-6s (unsaturated fats) are necessary, but most people already consume more than enough in processed and junk foods, so you don't need to look for another source. To eat for better sleep, enjoy a moderate amount of some of these foods every day: wild-caught salmon, mackerel, sardines, anchovies, chia seeds, flaxseeds, sunflower seeds, olive oil, almond oil, avocado oil, peanut oil, almonds, cashews, and walnuts.

Foods with tryptophan help make you feel sleepy. Known as L-tryptophan, it is an amino acid only found in food or supplements. It helps reduce anxiety and relax muscles. Tryptophan also pairs well with carbohydrates. The combination stimulates insulin and that, in turn, helps the tryptophan to be absorbed in the brain, promoting sleep. Foods high in this essential amino acid are milk, turkey, canned tuna, Cheddar cheese, oats, fruit, whole-wheat bread, dark chocolate, nuts, and seeds. Have a small amount, equivalent to a small handful.

Drink something warm and calming. A cup of chamomile or valerian root tea before bed will relax you. Have a small cup (just 10 ounces [296 ml] or so), so your bladder won't feel full. Or drink Golden Milk (page 25) with a pinch of ground nutmeg. Historically, this aromatic spice is said to increase sleepiness. Drink it about a half hour before bed. Use real dairy (goat or cow) or go with a plant-based milk if that suits your gut better.

Doshas and Appetite

Each dosha has a different hunger level. Pittas are usually ravenous in the morning and at mealtimes. Vata is hungry but easily gets distracted and forgets to eat or snacks on small bites throughout the day. Kapha isn't really hungry but eats because the clock says so, and they've heard that breakfast is the most important meal of the day, and they don't want to miss it. In the Kapha mind, even if they are not hungry, breakfast is at 8 a.m., lunch is at noon, and dinner is at 6 p.m.

It's important to be aware of your appetite, to nourish yourself properly throughout the day, and to leave time for the digestive process in the evening. When you pay attention, you'll see that what, how much, and when you eat during the day plays a key role in how you sleep at night. I tell my clients to focus on their hunger level and eat when they feel hungry. Kapha might eat at 10 a.m. or not at all. For Pitta, it's 7 a.m. or soon after they wake up. Vata needs to set a schedule and check in with themselves so they don't forget.

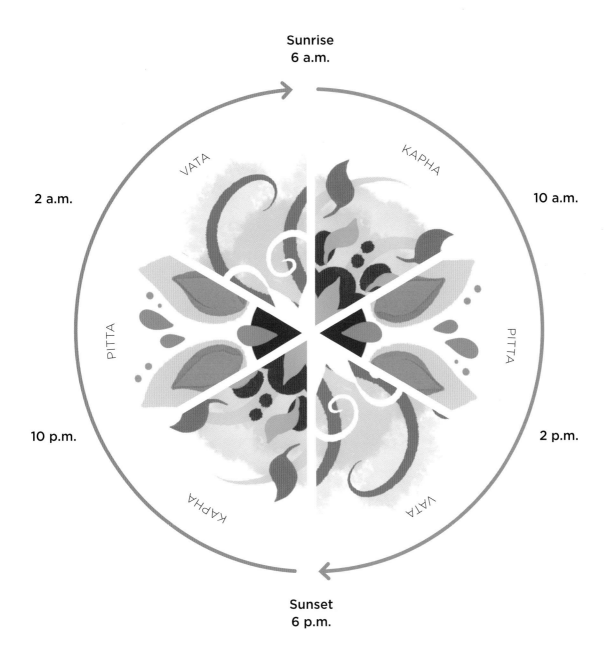

Sunrise
6 a.m.

VATA

KAPHA

2 a.m.

10 a.m.

PITTA

PITTA

10 p.m.

2 p.m.

KAPHA

VATA

Sunset
6 p.m.

What and When to Eat

The New York Times reported that researchers found that eating a diet high in sugar, saturated fat, and processed carbohydrates disrupts sleep. Eating more plants, fiber, and foods rich in unsaturated fat (such as nuts, olive oil, fish, and avocados) has the opposite effect, promoting sound sleep.

Whatever time of day it is for you, breakfast does not need to be a feast—just enough to get you going. Think real food, but not too much. A small bowl of whatever you choose—oatmeal, avocado, tofu, eggs over rice, toast, fruit, or soup—is a good option. A granola bar, raw bar, or bar of any kind is not a good choice. It is not food (it's highly processed) and will just leave you unsatisfied and unnourished.

The heaviest/largest meal of the day, according to Ayurveda, is lunch. Enjoy it sometime between 10 a.m. and 2 p.m., when the sun is highest in the sky. Lunch coincides with Pitta time of day (details on page 23), and it helps you metabolize food intake. This hearty meal will sustain you through the rest of the day, leaving you wanting just a small meal as the day winds down. A satisfying meal is a combination of carbs, protein, fiber, and fat. Cooked food is always better than raw.

Between 5 p.m. and 7 p.m., have a light, easy-to-digest supper. Soup, steamed veggies, a bit of protein, and some carbs and fat (good oils such as olive, ghee, sesame, walnut, or avocado) will get you through the night. Complex carbohydrates equal better sleep. Forget processed food completely, especially at dinner, as it will totally disturb the digestive process and disrupt your sleep. The added chemicals are impossible to digest and impede the process of absorbing nutrients.

End the evening with a cup of herbal tea or Golden Milk (page 25) (with or without dairy, depending on your preference). Give yourself at least 3 hours after eating before you go to sleep (10 p.m. at the latest) and sip your tea right up until you turn out the lights.

Sleepy Time Golden Milk

While you sip, read something soothing, listen to a guided meditation or some music, or gaze into the distance and relax. The act of holding a warm mug in your hands is a calming ritual. Inhale deeply, enjoy the rich scent of the spices, and get ready for sleep.

- 1 cup (235 ml) whole (goat or cow) milk or plant milk
- 1 pinch ginger powder
- 1 pinch turmeric powder
- 1 pinch cinnamon
- 1 pinch nutmeg
- 1 teaspoon ghee
- 1 teaspoon jaggery, Sucanat, or Florida crystals (optional)

Whisk all the ingredients together in a small pot. Bring to a boil over medium-high heat, then quickly take off the heat. Pour the Golden Milk into a mug and settle into bed to enjoy.

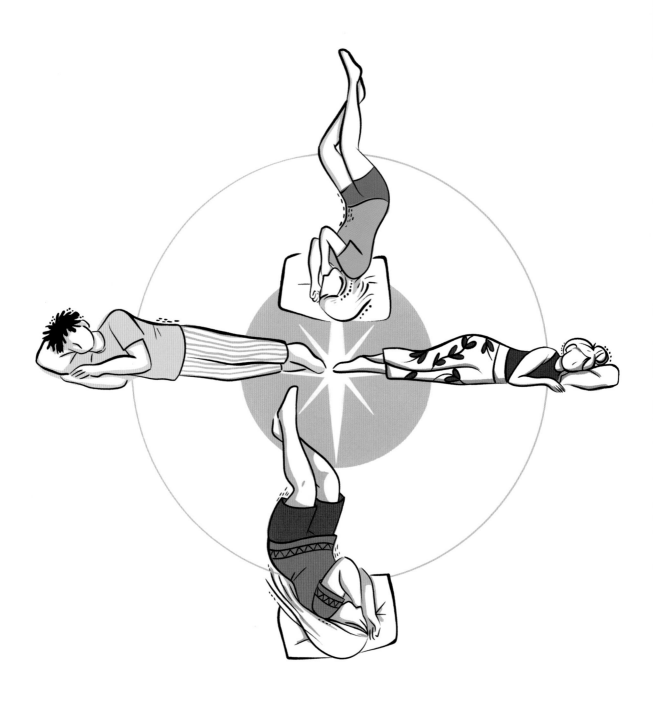

LIFESTYLE: CREATING A RESTFUL SPACE

Position the head of your bed to face any direction *except* north. According to Vastu Shastra (Vedic precursor to Feng Shui, the art and science of placement, design, and direction), the head ideally would be to the south or west, which are said to be the directions best suited to promoting rest and relaxation based on magnetic and astrological alignments, with the feet facing north or east. If possible, the bedroom is set in the southwest corner of the house. If you can't change the direction of your bed, try sleeping at the opposite end to reposition head and feet.

Keep the space under your bed clear. Ancient beliefs say the soul travels around the bed at night but, if there are obstacles, it cannot complete its task and becomes agitated. Remove any boxes, storage, or clutter, and let your soul roam free. While you are at it, clear your night table off. Have only the essentials. Less clutter creates a calmer, more settled space. And avoid having a mirror at the foot of the bed: The soul might be startled.

Make the room dark, cool, and fresh. Begin lowering the lights in the house at sunset so that your body will start its natural production of melatonin, the sleep hormone. Bright lights keep this hormone from secreting into the brain. We sleep best between 62°F and 68°F (17°C to 20°C). If you have a bed partner who wants it warmer, set a small fan or air cooler on your side of the bed and open a window a bit to let in fresh air. The good bacteria and oxygen from outside air clear the lungs of toxins.

Night Mode

Consider removing electronics from your room. For many of us, this may sound extreme or unnecessary, but it matters. Electronics emit electromagnetic frequencies (EMF) that may disrupt your brain waves—and they also remind us of activities and work. One of the best things you can do to improve sleep hygiene is to keep the computer, television, tablets, and phones out of the bedroom (or at least keep them as far away from the bed as possible). Even in airplane mode, most don't turn off completely.

Write in a Journal Before Bed

Keeping a journal will help you let go of nagging thoughts, plans, and ideas that are on your mind. Leave them in a journal so they won't wake you up.

If you must look at a screen, put it in night mode, lower the brightness, or wear amber-colored glasses to block blue light. Don't read upsetting emails or address difficult issues in the hours before bedtime. If you have a TV in your room, cover it with a piece of fabric before sleep and unplug it.

APOTHECARY: SLEEPY TIME AIDS

- Bhringaraj oil. This Ayurvedic herbal-infused oil helps calm the nervous system and cool the body. Before bed, rub a dime-sized amount into your scalp and a bit more to cover the soles of your feet. Put socks on and a towel on your pillow, if needed.

- Valerian root, chamomile, and skullcap. These herbs are found in Ayurvedic sleep formulas and are useful for drifting off to sleep. Take one or two tablets about a half hour before bed. Tea can be prepared from these leaves. Caution: Do not use these formulas if you are pregnant.

- Lavender and nutmeg oil. Apply directly to the skin with a carrier oil, such almond, sesame, or jojoba. Take a drop or two of one or the other; rub it into your forehead and pulse points.

- Melatonin. This supplement is great to use if you are trying to get to bed earlier or if you have jet lag. Only use it for a short period to regulate and reset your sleep patterns. Typical amounts are between 0.05 and 5 milligrams about one hour before bed. Check with your physician to ensure it is safe for you.

Put Me to Bed Bathing Routine

For a relaxing bath to prepare you for restful sleep, look to Epsom salts and lavender essential oil. Enjoy a cup of chamomile or lavender tea while relaxing in the bath.

- 2 cups (448 g) Epsom salts
- 10 to 15 drops lavender oil
- Vata-calming oil, such as sesame seed or almond oil

Fill a tub with hot water. Add the Epsom salts and oil. Rest in the bath for about 20 minutes. Exit the tub and pat dry. Apply a small amount of oil to your entire body. Allow the oil to absorb fully before dressing. The simple act of slowly massaging your limbs, belly, neck, and scalp allows the mind and body to let go and deeply relax.

If you don't have time for a bath, try warming up the oil and massaging the whole body, or even just the joints, belly, scalp, and soles of the feet. The nervous system responds by releasing tension and allowing you to rest more deeply.

Condition: Insomnia

If you wake in the middle of the night, note the time. We have doshic times of day and night. The hour when you wake up and can't fall back to sleep will correlate with a doshic cycle. If you consistently wake up before 2 a.m., this is the Pitta phase. If you wake between 2 a.m. and 6 a.m., this is the Vata stage. Kapha time is 6 a.m. to 10 a.m.

PITTA TIME

A person who can't fall asleep or who wakes up during Pitta time (10 p.m. to 2 a.m.) is usually dealing with unfinished business, problem solving, resentments, blame, aggravation, and frustration. Pitta becomes impatient and upset with themselves or blames others for being awake and not being able to go back to sleep. They will try to power through it, telling themselves they don't need any more sleep. This leaves them hot and bothered. When you wake in this time frame, try any of the following strategies.

Food

- Avoid hot, spicy food during the day but especially in the evening meal. Stick to a balanced mix of mild spices with protein, fiber, carbs, and fat.

- Red wine increases heat. If an alcoholic drink is needed, have a beer or a white wine. Or skip altogether and enjoy calming herbal tea blends.

Lifestyle

- Turn on a dim light; red or yellow light bulbs are best. Try journaling thoughts onto the page and leave them there.

- Listen to calming music, chants, or mantras. If using a phone or tablet, set a timer for it to turn off. Try a podcast to lull you back to sleep.

- Practice cooling *sheetali* breathing (page 174).

- Keep the room cool. Use a fan if needed.

- Wear a lightweight, organic cotton nightshirt. Stick to cooling colors such as pastels, beige, white, blue, or green. Avoid red, orange, and black, as they are not conducive to good sleep.

- Keep a glass of water next to the bed and sip when you wake to avoid dehydration.

Apothecary

- Place a few drops of nutmeg or sandalwood oil on your forehead, on your pulse points, and at the base of your throat.
- Massage cooling Bhringaraj oil on your head and feet before bed. Pour a dime-sized amount into your hand, rub your palms together, and press into your scalp. Rub around your ears and neck, then use enough to cover your toes and feet and massage in deeply.

VATA TIME

When you wake up in Vata time (2 a.m. to 6 a.m.), the mind ruminates on past events, reviewing and lamenting past experiences, worrying about the future, and being anxious about the present. The chatter in the head may be difficult to quiet down. Vata will feel wide awake, hopeless that they will ever fall back to sleep, and may become sad or despondent. When you wake in this time frame, try any of the following strategies.

Food

- Hunger can wake Vata up at night and is the only dosha to benefit from a bit of food before bed. Try protein mixed with carbs, like a small baked potato with ghee, toast with butter, or a tablespoon (16 g) of nut butter.
- Stay hydrated by sipping some warm water before bed.

Lifestyle

- Sit up and put on a dim light; red or yellow light bulbs are best. Look around the room or outside, and allow yourself to come back to the present moment. Open a window to allow fresh air into the room to improve blood circulation and brain function.
- Write in a journal. Note the past, present, and future thoughts. Then leave them on the page.
- Practice alternate nostril breathing (page 175) to ground yourself and oxygenate the blood.
- Listen to a sleep meditation or podcast. Set a timer for the app to turn off.

- If you are in bed with another person, try asking them to hold you, or hold them for grounding. A pet is great for this, too. Even stroking another person or pet— skin to skin or skin to fur contact—is very soothing. If alone, cross your arms over your chest and rub the upper arms up and down. This calming practice increases serotonin, oxytocin, and dopamine.

- Get comfortable and snuggle down into bed. Repeat a soothing mantra such as "all is right with the world" or "deep sleep is here for me." Relax and let go.

- Any time of day or just before bed, practice Earthing. Sit or walk outside in bare feet on grass, sand, or dirt, for about 10 to 20 minutes. This will help to align your body's natural rhythm with the Earth and the seasons, helping to regulate your sleep, calm you, and help you be more in balance with the rhythms of nature.

- Wear organic cotton pajamas or a long nightgown to stay warm, and wear socks.

- Use earplugs to block out noises as Vata, a light sleeper, wakes up easily.

- Keep a glass of water next to the bed and sip when you wake to avoid dehydration.

Apothecary

- Rub a few drops of lavender or rose oil onto your pulse points at the wrist, behind the ears, and at the base of the throat.

- Massage Bhringaraj oil into your temples and around your ears.

- Press into the Marma points (see page 34) at the *Ajna* point, the third eye, which is between your eyebrows. Place a drop of nutmeg oil on the tip of the ring finger (the earth element). This can provide grounding. If you are feeling overheated, try any finger, except the thumb (fire). Place your finger on the point and hold for at least one minute, pressing just enough so that you feel it, but it doesn't hurt. It's a sensitive point.

- Other Marma points include the space between the second and third toes, on the sole of the foot, about one-third up from the heel (this point is effective for relieving headaches, leg pain, and stress in addition to insomnia), and the palm of the hand.

- Alternatively, you can place your finger on your skull, on a point corresponding to the frontal lobe, called the *Brahmarandhra* point. This point is eight fingers back from the brow point. Stack one hand on top of the other from the brow and up the forehead to find the point, usually 3 to 4 inches (7.5 to 10 cm) above the Ajna point. Nutmeg oil works well, as does *jatamamsi* oil, and can quiet the mind as well as emotional disruptions. Hold for at least 1 minute and remember to breathe deeply.

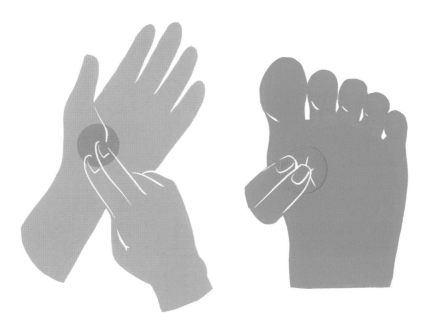

Put pressure on these Marma points: Apply medium pressure with the index and middle fingers (cooling air and space), for at least 30 seconds to the base of the thumb joint; then the base of the big toe joint. Use these two fingers to circle around the navel in a clockwise direction for at least 30 seconds.

Marma Therapy

Akin to acupressure, acutouch, and acupuncture, Marma therapy accesses the juncture between meridian points in the body that promote and amplify healing. In Marma, we use our fingers, a wooden pointer, or sometimes a tuning fork to create pressure and facilitate healing. Press the desired Marma point for one to two minutes, using medium, steady pressure.

The fingers play a major role when doing the ancient Ayurvedic therapy of Marma. Each finger is associated with one of the five elements.

- The thumb represents fire.
- The index finger is air.
- The middle finger is space.
- The ring finger is earth.
- The pinky represents water.

Become familiar with the power of the elements that you hold in your hands, as well as methods to balance physical and even emotional pain.

Ajna or Sthapani

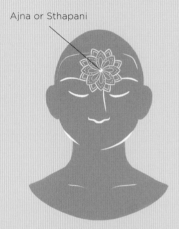

- If you have a sharp, hot headache, don't use your thumb (fire) to rub your temples. Apply air (index), space (middle), or water (pinky) to help balance the heat.
- If you have achy, dull pain in your knee, apply light pressure with your thumb to heat it up and get the stagnation and blood moving.
- If insomnia is an issue, apply pressure to the palm of your hand with your ring finger for grounding.
- When feeling dull and lethargic, use the index and middle fingers at the base of your skull, behind your ears to wake you up.

Brahmarandhra

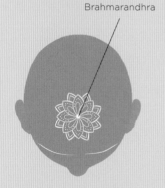

KAPHA TIME

Kapha dosha could be called the cozy dosha. They love to cuddle, snuggle, and stay in bed wrapped up in a warm blanket. They nest. Kapha time of day is 6 a.m. to 10 a.m. You may notice if you wake up around 6 a.m. or 6:30 a.m., you feel wide awake and ready to go, just coming off Vata time. But someone who is primarily Kapha dosha, or has been ill or depressed, or went to bed late, might prefer to roll over and try to sleep for a few more hours. Upon waking up at 8 a.m., 9 a.m., or 10 a.m., they will feel groggy or lethargic. Kapha time is that slow time of day when we should ready ourselves for action and activity. Try some of these remedies to help you shake off that sleepy feeling and find more energy.

Food

- Eat a light dinner and don't consume anything except for herbal tea after 6 p.m. or 7 p.m. at the latest. This is supremely important: it will help you fall asleep earlier and be hungrier in the morning.

- Don't drink alcohol, especially in the evening. Opt for herbal tea instead. Even Golden Milk might be too heavy. Less dairy is better, so if you are craving Golden Milk (page 25), enjoy a nondairy option, such as hemp milk, and even add a splash of hot water.

- Avoid heavy food (fast, fried, fatty, oily, sweet, and dairy) during the day. These increase the weight of Kapha in the mind and body. Eat less sweet, salty, and sour foods, and choose more bitter, pungent, and astringent ones. Think: less pasta, sugar, wheat, dairy, and nuts; more beans, whole grains, fresh fruit, greens, and seeds.

- Try intermittent fasting. Have your last meal of the day by 5 p.m. or 6 p.m., then fast for about 15 hours and have your next meal at 8 a.m. or 9 a.m. This is a great way to detox, allow the digestive system to rest, and use up stored sources of energy (undigested food). That metabolic rest will help you sleep more deeply and wake up earlier, refreshed and rejuvenated.

- Enjoy coffee, green tea, or black tea in the morning. A bit of caffeine helps to get Kapha moving: 1 to 3 cups (237 to 710 ml) is fine. Avoid using dairy cream and sugar, and don't have caffeine after 2 p.m.

Lifestyle

- Wear an unrestrictive nightshirt made of organic cotton. Pastel, light green, yellow, and orange are best for Kapha sleep. If you feel cold or if you oil your feet before bed, wear socks.

- Get up when the sun rises. Waking naturally without an alarm is the best way to reset your sleep cycle. Sleep with a window and shades open just enough to allow the air and sun to come in. If you live in an area where the sun rises late, or if you do not have a window that lets light in, purchase a sunrise lamp, which will slowly illuminate to wake you at sunrise.

- Exercise for at least 30 minutes a day. For the greatest benefits, do a mix of aerobic exercises, stretching, and strength training throughout the week. Before bed, do a series of stretches and micro-movements, such as ankle and wrist rotations, seated twists, toe touches, and arm extensions high above your head with your back slightly arched. Some balance poses, such as tree pose, and even just standing on one foot help to balance both hemispheres of the brain before sleep. Hold your poses for at least 10 seconds. If you can't balance for 10 seconds, work up to it; use a chair or wall for support until you can manage without.

- Begin your day with breath work. In the morning, a round of ten deep, rapid inhalations to the belly followed by full exhalations through the nose is enough to really wake you up. Take just a few minutes for some invigorating breath work like *Bhastrika* (page 176). Caution: Build up slowly and avoid altogether if you have high blood pressure or cardiac issues or if you are pregnant.

- Stretch to get the blood flowing. Forward bends are great for waking up the brain. Bend forward, grasp your elbows, and just hang for 10 or 20 seconds. Rise up slowly and raise your arms over your head and point your fingers toward the ceiling, shoulders down. Look up. And a few rounds of Sun Salutations (page 179) will definitely get the blood and breath moving!

Apothecary

- Melatonin taken 1 hour before bed will induce sleep and wear off naturally by the morning. It's best to speak to a doctor or Ayurvedic practitioner for a specific dose, though typical amounts are between 0.05 and 5 milligrams.

- Use Bhringaraj oil to relax at bedtime. Perform a massage on the scalp and feet to help ensure that you fall asleep early and feel rested when you rise early.

Condition: Sleep Apnea

Sleep apnea means cessation of breathing during sleep. In some cases, the breath will cease for several seconds, up to thirty times in one hour, leaving the sleeper gasping for breath and snoring loudly between bouts of no breath at all. This occurs when the muscles in the throat become lax and there is a partial or complete occlusion of the airway. It is extremely disruptive for the sufferer, and it will keep a bed partner from being rested as well.

Good sleep is one of the main indicators of overall health. A person who is constantly cycling between sleep, wake, breathing, and not breathing will not be at the top of their game. The lack of sleep may cause digestive issues, fogginess, day sleeping, and extreme exhaustion. Their entire being suffers because restorative sleep is not achievable.

TREATING SLEEP APNEA

The number one cause of sleep apnea is obesity. Other causes are smoking and incessant mouth breathing. There are several home remedies to ease the issue. If they do not work and you are still suffering after a few months, please see a physician to look for other underlying causes. These remedies will also work for snoring.

Food

- Eat a Kapha-reducing diet. This means avoiding all dairy, wheat, and sugar—and I really mean *avoid* it. Take at least thirty days to see the results and continue as needed. This alone could cure you. Sustain this diet until you are at a normal weight for your height and dosha. See page 111 for details.

- Use a spice mixture of ginger, turmeric, and black pepper. Mix 1 tablespoon (15 g) of each in a jar and add it to all of your savory food.

- Do not overeat. Your two or three meals a day should be about two handfuls of food. Stop eating at least 3 hours before bed and enjoy a Cumin-Coriander-Fennel (CCF) tea (page 38) or licorice tea (page 38) to aid digestion.

- Avoid coffee, tea, and caffeinated drinks after 12 p.m. You may be tempted to drink coffee because you are sleepy, but don't.

- Do not drink alcohol. The effects of drinking, especially as the alcohol wears off, disturb sleep and breathing.

Lifestyle

- Get regular exercise every day. If you are overweight, try walking every day for 15 or 20 minutes, building up to longer walks. Add in strength training; hand weights are great and convenient. Then add in stretching, like yoga. The more you move, the more you will want to move! Every little bit counts, so begin with what you are comfortable with and slowly increase when you feel ready. The benefits of exercise go way beyond the body. As you move, you detox the lymphatic system, pushing toxins out and allowing the happy hormones, such as serotonin and oxytocin, to reach the brain. Runner's high is a real thing!

Digestive Teas

Cumin-Coriander-Fennel (CCF) tea is easy to make and can aid a sluggish digestive system. Add ½ teaspoon each of cumin, coriander, and fennel seeds to 12 ounces (355 ml) of hot water. Steep for 10 minutes. Strain and enjoy.

Licorice tea is another simple way to help your digestion. Add ¼ to ½ teaspoon of licorice to 12 ounces (355 ml) of hot water. Steep for about 5 minutes. Caution: Don't take licorice if you are pregnant.

- Improve air quality. Keep your bedroom well humidified, using a humidifier if needed. Open windows to bring in healing oxygen and beneficial bacteria. Quit smoking, and do not be around anyone who smokes.

- Make your body comfortable for sleep. Sleep on your left side: This supports your organs and may help the flap in the back of the throat stay open. Prop your head up when you go to sleep, either using extra pillows, or if you have a bed with an adjustable frame, raising the head up to a comfortable level.

- Get new pillows, sheets, and a mattress cover. Hypoallergenic, organic bed coverings may help you breathe easier and block irritants such as dust mites. Use only natural cleaning products in your house, including detergents, cleaners, and dusters.

- Practice alternate nostril breathing (page 175) or boxed breathing (page 177) to learn how to breathe deeply through your nose. You may feel that you are clogged and not getting enough air; stay with it and your nasal passages eventually will open up.

Apothecary

- Before bed, gargle with either warm water or 1 tablespoon (15 ml) of warm sesame seed oil. This will coat the throat and relieve feelings of dryness.

- Mix ¼ teaspoon pippali powder with 1 teaspoon raw, organic honey and lick off the spoon twice a day (morning and evening are best). Take every day for as long as needed. Pippali, also known as piper longum, is a fruit powder related to black pepper. It's hot and pungent, which helps to burn away toxins, stimulating digestion, clearing the lungs, and promoting easy breathing. You can find it online from Ayurvedic stores.

- Use nasya oil before bed. Coat the inside of your nostrils with three to five drops of the oil. Close the nostrils, pinch them, and take a deep sniff, releasing the nostrils and feeling the oil in the back of the throat. Nasya oil comes premixed with herbs that open the nasal passages and block toxins. The nourishing oils coat the tissues of the sinuses to keep them healthy and prepared to block invasions of allergens and environmental toxins. It's easy to find in health food stores or online. You can also use sesame seed oil or ghee in the same way.

Going Beyond the Usual

There is a study that shows that playing the didgeridoo might cure sleep apnea (pubmed.ncbi.nlm.nih.gov/16377643). It goes to reason that singing or playing any wind instrument might help to tone and strengthen the throat, enabling the epiglottis to stay in place for you to breathe normally without cessation. It's worth a try!

Learn exercises for your tongue, throat, jaw, and facial muscles, such as sticking your tongue out as far as you can for 5 seconds, sucking your tongue to the roof of your mouth and holding for 5 seconds, and pushing your tongue against your top teeth for 5 seconds (do five to ten times each). There are videos online with detailed instructions for sleep apnea exercises that are beneficial, such as Vik Veer's "Throat Exercises for Snoring and Sleep Apnoea" on YouTube.

If you are a mouth breather, learn techniques such as mouth taping to encourage breathing through the nose. Use only tape designed for this practice and speak with your practitioner or doctor about it. Use breathing strips on your nose to keep the nasal passages open.

Condition: Nightmares

Nightmares occur more frequently in childhood, but adults are visited by them as well. Dreams, according to Ayurveda, are dosha-specific, which is both fascinating and helpful. If one of your doshas is extremely out of balance, it may show up in your dreams or nightmares, giving you a clue where you might need to focus your attention in creating a healthier lifestyle.

VATA DREAMS

Vata dreams involve flying, running, moving fast, confusion, anxiety, and worry. In a Vata-type dream, the person may find themselves falling, being chased, or being attacked without knowing why or where to turn for help. Air, space, and movement figure prominently. Vata may not remember their dreams when they wake up, but they usually recall feelings and emotions of being scared and confused.

PITTA DREAMS

Pitta is often running, fighting, or involved in a great challenge or competition. Sometimes violent acts, such as combat or street fighting, will take over the dreams. They usually are trying to figure a way out, and to understand what is going on. They are frustrated and impatient at not finding a solution or winning. These dreams can involve fire, intense heat, lightning, and storms. Pittas usually have vivid recall of details and may wake up disturbed and angry.

KAPHA DREAMS

Kapha dreams are watery and sensual. Streets turn into rivers and oceans swell up to encompass everything. Kapha may swim to safety, find that they cannot get out of the water, or drown. Food has a prominent role, specifically sweet foods such as cakes, cookies, and candy. They may stuff their mouths uncontrollably or search for food. Kapha will remember the dreams, and bad dreams may leave them feeling guilty and sad.

Food

- For Vata dreams: If you are having confusing, unsettling dreams, eat a handful of nuts or a small bowl of popcorn with ghee or olive oil before bed. Drink warm milk or Golden Milk (page 25) with ghee.

- For Pitta dreams: If you have violent, scary dreams, have some coconut water or CCF tea (page 38) before bed. Or try a few ounces of dark chocolate.

- For Kapha dreams: Do not eat after 7 p.m. A cup of CCF tea (page 38) will help to settle fears in dreams.

Lifestyle

- Avoid upsetting tasks in the evening. Leave paying bills, balancing your checkbook, or having difficult conversations for daytime.

- Don't watch scary or intense movies or TV shows in the evening. Save them for a rainy Sunday afternoon. Definitely stay away from the news. Watch comedies, light dramas, or uplifting documentaries. Listening to soothing music is a good option.

- Enjoy comforting, enjoyable books, articles, or podcasts. Have some guided meditations on hand for sleep and listen in bed.

- Keep a journal at your bedside and jot down any thoughts that are swirling in your mind as you prepare for sleep. If you wake up disturbed in the night, jot it down and leave it on the page.

- Practice alternate nostril (page 175) or boxed breathing (page 177) when you get into bed. It will settle you down, quiet the sympathetic nervous system (the fight-or-flight reaction), and activate the parasympathetic nervous system, which relaxes the body and mind.

Apothecary

- Take two ashwagandha tablets or drink ¼ teaspoon of the powder in warm water before bed. This will relax you and promote restful sleep.

- Drink valerian root tea 1 hour before bed. Valerian is an ancient plant that has been used to promote sleep for centuries. If you are taking other sleep aids, check with your doctor before taking. You can buy leaves or powder. Use about ½ teaspoon per 12 ounces (355 ml) of water, and steep for 10 minutes. There are plenty of blends on the market for sleep with valerian, lavender, and chamomile.

- Place a few drops of lavender essential oil on your pillow. The nanoparticles will enter your nasal passages and your bloodstream to help you drift off and, hopefully, stay sleeping through the night.

- Keep a window open a bit for fresh air to keep you oxygenated and refreshed during the night.

- Do *abhyanga* massage (page 174) before bed, with just enough oil to do long, deep strokes.

- Use Bhringaraj oil on your feet and scalp before going to sleep. This will help keep you cool and calm.

Winding Down

Whether you struggle to get good sleep or you want to benefit from more restful, restorative sleep, know that it may take some trial and error to find the right fit for you. Take your time and create your own personal routine. Getting frustrated or impatient (Pitta qualities) only adds to the problem.

Try looking at the qualities of Kapha dosha to invite better sleep into your life. Kapha is sedentary, sensual, caring, and patient. Clean, soft sheets, a warm comforter, and loose-fitting bedclothes create a sweet sleep space. Fill your senses with lavender oil on the body or sheets and drink warm milk with ghee, nutmeg, and turmeric. Take the time for a warm bath and then a slow massage with vanilla-scented oil.

Try just one or two suggestions at a time, and add more as you find your way to what works for you. It took years to create your current habits, so be patient and gentle with yourself as you embark on a new lifestyle. Slow and steady creates new habits that will benefit you for a lifetime.

Remember that when and what we eat plays such a huge role in how we sleep and this may be the first time you have thought about how food affects your sleep. Pay attention to your hunger level so that you manage your meals for optimal sleep. Pitta might be hungry, so have more hearty foods earlier in the day. Vata may need to eat smaller, more frequent meals. Eat three meals a day, and a light dinner at least 3 hours before bed. If you are primarily Kapha dosha, you might find that two meals are enough, especially in spring and summer.

Many days, especially in summer when *agni* (digestive fire) is low, I'm not hungry, so I eat a healthy meal around 10 a.m. or 11 a.m. Sometimes it's just a green veggie juice or a fruit smoothie with oat milk, berries, and protein powder. I have another meal when I'm hungry around 4 p.m. or 5 p.m. This is a great routine in summer for Kapha or if you are trying to lose weight. Winter breakfast, or the first meal of the day, is more substantial, such as oatmeal with flaxseeds and ghee, cornmeal pancakes, or a quinoa bowl with nuts, ghee, and cooked greens. Play with your meal schedule to find what works best.

As one of the main pillars of Ayurveda, sleep determines overall health and well-being, mentally and physically. It simply cannot be overestimated how important it is. My suggestion to you is if you are struggling with other health issues, try focusing on your sleep first. It's terribly difficult to feel well and make good decisions when your sleep is not good.

I've gone through several periods in my life when I felt off, slightly depressed, angry, unfocused, and sad. Stepping back and looking at my daily routine helped me put things into focus. Almost always, my sleep routine was off, staying up too late, eating a large meal at dinner, snacking in the evening, drinking alcohol, or watching or reading news before bed. All of that contributed to poor sleep, which led to unhappy days. If you make the changes outlined in this chapter, it will help you improve your sleep, your digestion, your decision-making, and your mood. And with that, you will start to feel healthier and happier and be more productive. Just a few good nights can be enough to get you on the path to feeling better. Try it.

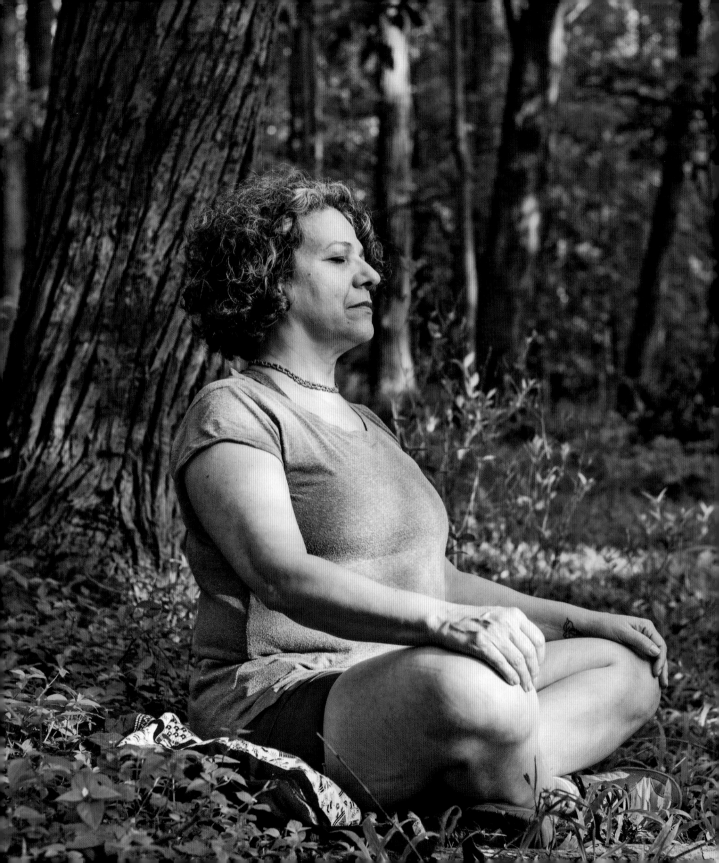

2

Pain:
Mind and Body Relief

Ayurveda says pain has a message: It's knocking us on the head, or tripping us over, begging us to listen closely. "Mind over matter" is one age-old belief system that says you can think your way out of pain. In this chapter, we will talk about different approaches to this: meditation, mindfulness, and breath work. You'll practice remedies and methods *before* you are suffering, and you'll learn effective ways to respond when pain arises. By being mindful, you'll notice when pain begins as a tiny seed of discomfort. Then you can address it right away, before the pain establishes roots, spreads, and invades the body.

Doshic Responses to Pain

We all have pain at some time or another. While you may have pain due to an injury, degeneration of the tissues, aging, or nutritional deficiencies, pain has something to tell you. Maybe it's that you are overusing a body part (repetitive motion); not sleeping well; not eating or hydrating properly; not paying attention to your body; experiencing shallow breathing; suppressing emotions, needs and desires, or natural urges. Pain says *pay attention*.

Pain and pain relief are individual, especially when you look at it through the lens of the doshas. We each experience pain differently, as some have a higher tolerance for aches and pains than others. Begin self-care and healing by being aware of your doshic response to pain. Vata dosha can get very upset and disoriented by pain and have a hard time articulating what is wrong. Pitta may be angry and frustrated, trying to work through it on their own without proper rest and care, causing more damage. Kapha would rather not bother or upset anyone else, so they often keep illnesses secret. Kapha and Pitta might ignore or brush off pain until it is deeply rooted and nearly too late for repair.

Pain is always associated with the dosha Vata. Vata, as you recall, is like the wind. It spreads and is pervasive, mobile, changeable. So, while you may not be a predominantly Vata person, the pain you feel is caused by excess Vata in certain areas of the body, behaving in a way that causes discomfort. The drying attributes of Vata may cause a loss of synovial fluid and lubrication of the joints, resulting in arthritis or inflammation, hindering the repair of muscles and tissues and natural detoxification.

Preventing and Managing All Types of Pain

Chronic inflammation is the root cause of many illnesses and pains. Movement and sleep are equally important so that the body has time to repair itself. Remember "move it or lose it" holds true in most situations. Movement keeps the joints lubricated and helps you avoid additional stiffness. Mobility may be limited, but it is good to try to move either on your own or with a yoga therapist or physical therapist.

FOOD: EATING TO REDUCE PAIN

- Eat an anti-inflammatory diet. Incorporating whole foods into your diet will leave you feeling fully nourished and satisfied. Your daily intake should look like a rainbow.

- Use more spices in your food, especially turmeric and ginger. Sauté spices in a bit of oil to activate their healing properties, and add them to your beans, grains, or greens. It's said that ½ teaspoon of turmeric a day is ideal to reduce inflammation in the entire body.

- It's called junk food for a reason. Avoid soda and sugary drinks and foods. Avoid all fast food, grilled (foods prepared over high, searing heat can have cancer-causing chemicals like acrylamide) and fried foods, and processed snacks, including bars, granola, and power drinks.

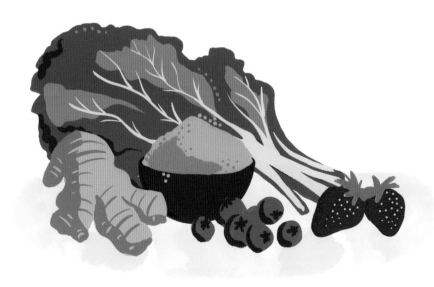

Think of Your Diet as a Pyramid

At the wide base, you should have fruits, berries, leafy greens, and veggies.

Then go for beans, lentils, black-eyed peas, and hummus.

Include whole grains (e.g., millet, quinoa, brown or basmati rice, oats, and barley) and pasta.

Add some healthy fats, such as olive oil and ghee.

Eat nuts, especially walnuts. (I like to call walnuts vegetarian salmon, as they are packed with omega-3 fatty acids.)

Eat avocados and seeds (e.g., pumpkin, sunflower, hemp, and freshly ground flaxseeds).

In moderation, enjoy oily fish (e.g., herring, sardines, salmon, and cod), tofu and soy products, cooked mushrooms, eggs, poultry, fresh cheese, and plain whole-fat yogurt.

Have a sweet tooth? Enjoy 1 to 2 ounces (28 to 55 g) of dark chocolate a day (over 70 percent cacao).

Sip warm or room temperature water throughout the day. Drink white or green tea instead of coffee, and only have red wine occasionally.

LIFESTYLE: PRIORITIZING SELF-CARE PRACTICES

Get moderate exercise in your daily routine. This could mean a 10- or 20-minute walk, some stretching, gentle twists, forward bends, micro-movements, swimming, or working out with light weights. If you're bed-bound or have trouble standing or walking, try bed yoga or chair yoga (page 180), like leg lifts, arm raises, seated forward bends, and stretching the arms above your head. Seated twists are great as well. Move however and whatever you are able to.

Meditate for 10 to 30 minutes a day. Use guided meditations for pain relief: Sit or lie down in a comfortable position, and breathe deeply through your nose. Listen as you are guided to work with the pain by visualizing, accepting, and letting go of the outcome.

Go to a doctor or health professional when you need to. Some of us are inclined to avoid asking for help, but the truth is we may not fully understand pain and how to treat it. Sometimes we need a professional. Functional medicine doctors and other alternative and complementary medicine professionals offer many holistic and other forms of relief. Sometimes it takes a combination of Western and Eastern medicine to heal.

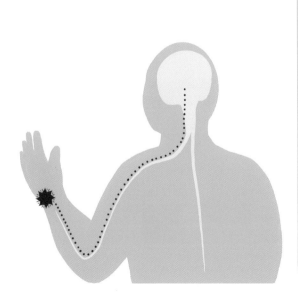

Tune In to Your Body

A body scan is a great way to concentrate on different parts of your body. Start at your feet and move your attention up your body, finishing at the top of your head. As you do this, name each body part as you pass through it, noticing all the areas of your body where you don't feel pain. Linger in those areas and allow the lack of pain to spread. To expand on this practice, try my meditation for working with pain on page 60.

Increase hobbies or other activities to get your mind off the pain. If you can, volunteer with people or animals in need. Giving your time to others is an incredibly powerful way to lessen your focus on your own problems. Find a creative release such as painting, journaling, writing to prompts, or listening to music. Fill your field of awareness with beauty to feed your senses. Flowers, colorful scarves, music, scents, soft blankets, and clothes create an atmosphere of healing and happiness.

APOTHECARY: NATURAL PAIN RELIEVERS

Turmeric. If you do not eat turmeric daily, take a supplement. Be sure it's the whole turmeric root (not the isolate curcumin); it works better just as nature created it. Take one or two tablets a day with food and some fat, or use at least ½ to 1 teaspoon a day in your cooking. To release the full potential of turmeric, sauté it in a high-heat oil like ghee or coconut oil before adding it to your food.

Ginger. Add ginger to your daily diet in any way you prefer: Drink 2 to 3 cups (480 to 720 ml) of ginger tea throughout the day. Make ginger water by adding a few slices of ginger to a cup of hot water. Use more fresh ginger or powdered ginger in cooking. One teaspoon a day is a good measure.

Guggulu, boswellia, guduchi, and pippali. Vata-reducing and balancing supplements may provide pain relief. Find Ayurveda brands for pain relief that contain these herbs and more. Usually, take one to two tablets a day before food. For chronic pain, take two tablets once a day, as needed.

Abhyanga body massage. See page 174 for massage instructions. Perform this massage every day. If you cannot do a full massage, concentrate on the painful areas and the joints where toxins accumulate.

Mahanarayan oil. Use this for pain relief, especially of the joints. Adding camphor or eucalyptus oil, like Tiger Balm liniment, enhances its qualities. Warm the oil under hot water, then apply liberally to the painful areas, using as deep a massage as possible, in circular motions on the joints and up and down on long bones.

Condition: Headache

You probably have experienced many types of headaches in your life. Some are hot and pounding, others dull and throbbing. Hormonal changes, such as menstruation, can bring on a nauseating headache. Dehydration and not eating enough create their own forms of headaches.

When one strikes, take a moment to determine what is going on. Are you hungry or thirsty? Have you been shallow breathing? You can remedy that pretty fast. Other types of headaches may need deeper inquiry. I list types of headaches here that are related to specific doshas. Disregard *your* specific dosha and look at the quality of the pain itself. It's speaking to you about something that needs to be addressed. Follow the guidelines for the pain you are experiencing, which can be remedied by appeasing a doshic imbalance.

VATA HEADACHES

Stress, exhaustion, anxiety, and worry types of headaches are specifically related to Vata dosha.

Food

- Eat and drink. One of the main causes for a Vata-type headache is not eating or drinking. Stay on a three-meal-a-day schedule, setting an alarm to remind you if necessary. Eat enough at each meal to feel satisfied, about two-thirds the size of your stomach, which is two handfuls of food.
- Drink warm beverages throughout the day.

Lifestyle

- Stay warm. Wear layers so you can adjust as needed.
- Always wear a scarf and hat in cool weather.

Apothecary

- Calamus oil is calming, with a scent similar to cinnamon and a slight tranquilizing effect. Massage your neck, scalp, and shoulders with it. Always use a diluted blend and avoid during pregnancy.

- Haritaki powder is a dried fruit powder, widely available online. Take ¼ to ½ teaspoon in warm water.

- Oil nasal passages with sesame seed oil or nasya oil once or twice a day. Nasya oil, which is easy to find in health food stores and online, lubricates the nasal passages and sinuses, blocking environmental toxins and reducing inflammation. You can put two to three drops in each nostril or put the oil on your pinky and swish it around the nasal passages to coat thoroughly. Apply as needed.

- Use Marma point therapy: Gently squeeze the outer rims of the ears down to the lobe, then pull slightly down on the lobe. Do this four to six times. Press the ear flaps in with the index fingers (as if blocking noise) and hold for 30 seconds.

PITTA HEADACHES

Burning sensation in the temples, sensitivity to light, and sharp head and neck pain are results of a Pitta headache.

Food

- Cool down with coconut water and Pitta-pacifying foods such as cucumbers, ghee, and cool lime water.

- Stay hydrated by sipping room temperature water throughout the day.

Lifestyle

- Do several rounds of sheetali breathing (see page 174).

Apothecary

- Massage neck, shoulders, and scalp with coconut oil mixed with a few drops of sandalwood oil, eucalyptus oil, or rose oil.

- Use ghee in the nasal passages.

- Apply light pressure to the Marma points at the temples with either the index or pinky finger, for cooling. Slowly move your fingers in a clockwise direction for 30 seconds, while taking deep, even breaths through the nose.
- Lightly place the index finger to the third eye chakra point between the eyebrows, apply light pressure, and hold for 30 seconds to a minute. Breathe deeply through the nose.

KAPHA HEADACHES

Facial pain and sinus headaches are a result of too much Kapha.

Food

- Avoid dairy, fast food, fried food, and fatty food.

Lifestyle

- Exercise regularly to keep oxygen and blood moving through the body, dilating blood vessels and cleansing the tissues.
- Practice Bhastrika breathing (page 176) to encourage detoxification through the release of CO_2, which when built up can cause headaches and a variety of disorders.

Apothecary

- Use a neti pot (saline nasal wash) once or twice a day. See page 78 for details.
- Make a steam of 4 cups (960 ml) of hot water with three drops each of eucalyptus oil, lavender oil, and tea tree oil. Cover your head with a towel and place your face above the bowl at a comfortable distance over the steam. Breathe deeply through the nose. Do this for 10 minutes, once or twice a day.
- Apply light pressure to the Marma points just under each nostril with the index fingers, and hold for 30 seconds, breathing deeply though the nose. A drop or two of the above oils on your fingers is very effective.
- Use your index fingers to place light to medium pressure to the Marma points at the base of the skull where there are indentations, next to the spinal column. Hold for 30 seconds and release. Breathe deeply to the belly when applying pressure, relax your body, shoulders down, and exhale fully.

- A vigorous head massage will lessen headache pain by increasing circulation. Look online for the Indian form of head massage, or do it by massaging the scalp thoroughly with your fingertips, like washing your hair vigorously. Using the essential oils, mentioned on page 53, on your hands will give an extra boost to the massage.

Condition: Neck Pain

Pains in the neck and head may be caused by injuries, stress, tension, and repetitive motion. After an accident, we may be fearful of re-injuring ourselves, so we hold the area in a protective state. All of this increases stress and tension physically and mentally. The remedies involve healing from the inside out, fully engaging all the senses in the release of pain, stiffness, and aches.

FOOD

- Stay hydrated by drinking enough room temperature water throughout the day. Half your body weight in ounces is a good measure. So, if you weigh 150 pounds (68 kg), drink 75 ounces (2.2 L) of water a day.

LIFESTYLE

- Use meditation techniques (page 60) regularly to reduce pain by learning to recognize where the pain is coming from, why it is appearing, and what emotions arise.

- Practice deep breathing. Inhale through the nose to the belly, to the count of four. Hold for 4 seconds, then exhale through the nose 4 seconds. Hold at the end of the exhale for four. Do this five to ten times in a row, whenever needed. When you feel ready, increase to 6 then 8 seconds. Deep breathing activates the vagus nerve, alleviating tension and flooding the body with calm.

- Do small movements throughout the day to increase blood flow. Notice how you hold your phone to your ear and how you sit at the computer or while reading. Adjust yourself frequently. Look up from your work and gaze off into the distance once an hour, for at least 30 seconds. Take a minute or two to look out a window for maximum benefit. Do head circles, gently circling from left to right, chin to chest, several times a day—not just when it hurts.

APOTHECARY

- Massage neck and shoulders with an oil blend made of two to three drops of eucalyptus, cinnamon, and peppermint oils in 2 to 3 ounces (60 to 90 ml) of a base oil such as sesame or jojoba. Or use Tiger Balm liniment. Avoid the eyes.

Condition: Joint Pain/Arthritis

One who is primarily Vata dosha often displays dryness in their joints, a lack of synovial fluid. Kapha and Pitta normally have a good amount, but overuse and age can damage any dosha's joints. Pitta is typically quite athletic, which over the years can cause degeneration in the tissues and joints. Kapha dosha might be hyper-flexible and notice they are less so as they age. In addition, excess weight, which many a Kapha struggles with, can increase pressure on the lower back, knees, hips, ankles, and feet, resulting in pain. The following remedies address joint aches and pains for all doshas.

APOTHECARY

- *Dashamula* and *nirgundi* are two widely available Ayurvedic herbal powders to take for this type of pain. Mix ¼ teaspoon each in 2 to 4 ounces (60 to 120 ml) of warm water and drink before eating. Or look for an Ayurvedic pain relief blend such as Banyan's Joint Pain or Lifespan's Boswellia blend. Take two to four tablets a day as needed.

- Use mahanarayan oil with a few drops of Tiger Balm liniment, applied two to three times a day directly to the area of pain. Try this after a warm shower or bath and allow the oil to penetrate deeply, or place a warm cloth over the oiled area and rest.

- *Jambeera thailam* is excellent for shoulder and joint pain. This specialized oil is made from lemons and turmeric. Be aware that it will stain your clothes, but it is amazingly effective. Use a small amount, enough to cover the area with a thin sheen of oil, and massage in deeply to the joints. Allow it to dry before putting on clothes, or wear something that you don't mind staining yellow.

Condition: Muscle Aches and Strains

We all overdo it once in a while, or maybe under-do it. Muscles that aren't often engaged can act up when put into use. Nature presents challenges that create hazards in the body, such as shoveling the first snowfall or raking the yard in autumn. Having a year-round exercise routine, involving stretching and weight training that touches on each muscle group, will keep you limber and prepared for the bigger jobs. And don't discount stress and tension! Breathing deeply when you feel tightness on the mind and body, along with stretching, weights, and aerobics done a few times a week, every week of the year, is best. But when you find yourself with a strain or ache, the following remedies will help.

APOTHECARY

- Soak in a hot bath with 2 cups (448 g) of Epsom salts and ¼ cup (32 g) of powdered ginger.

- Apply the oils mahanarayan or jambeera for joint pain. Rest for a few days, using gentle movements to avoid stiffness.

Condition: Lower Back Pain

Most pain is related to Vata dosha. Nowhere else in the body is this more demonstrated than in the lower back. Vata has a spreading quality, allowing air and space to invade and spread until we can hardly find the point of origin. Lower back pain will affect most of us if we live long enough. It may be the result of overuse and abuse of the area from intense exercise, sitting too much, heavy lifting, an old mattress, constipation, or age. Additionally, Vata is cold: Exposure to cold weather; eating cold foods; and obesity, worry, anxiety, and fear all create stress and strain that can settle in the lower back.

To treat lower back pain efficiently, we need to calm Vata dosha. Keep the area warm, stay hydrated, stick to a routine of gentle movements, three meals a day, and 10 p.m. bedtime. Having a daily routine will actually ease your pain. We get stressed out when we don't know what is coming up next, where we are supposed to be, what we are going to do, and when. Write out a schedule and place it somewhere to see it regularly and you will be more at ease. You won't have to guess what to do. It's there for you as clear as day.

FOOD

- Eat a Vata-balancing diet. Avoid cold, dry, and raw food. Your gut needs to increase agni (digestive fire) to digest those foods, which takes the heat away from the lower back where you need it for circulation and healing.

- Encourage your body to use its natural healing powers by eating food that is easy to digest, such as soups and stews, white rice, steamed or roasted veggies, and oily fish such as salmon and mackerel. Use ghee, olive oil, and avocado oil in your cooking or add them to foods for more lubrication in the gut and joints. Avoid white sugar.

- Sip warm fluids throughout the day. One or two caffeinated drinks a day is okay, but don't overdo it. Coffee, black tea, and green tea are dehydrating, so be sure to have water to balance them out.

- Add fresh ginger and turmeric to your diet. Use 1 teaspoon each in your cooking every day. Or enjoy them as a tea; buy already blended or make your own (see below).

Teas

Ginger-turmeric tea is widely available, and for good reason! Ginger (*Zingiber officinale*) comes from the same flower as cardamom and turmeric. For centuries, ginger has been used in Asia not just for cooking, but as medicine too. Sore throats, digestive issues, and skin problems can all be healed with different applications of this root. It's also easy to grow if you live in a warm climate.

To make the tea, slice or grate a 1-inch (2.5-cm) piece of turmeric and a 1-inch (2.5-cm) piece of ginger into a small sauce pot. Add 12 to 16 ounces (355 to 475 ml) of water. Bring to a boil and simmer for about 10 minutes. Strain and drink. To sweeten, add raw honey.

LIFESTYLE

- Move your body regularly but not intensely. Swim. Walk or hike on flat ground. Lift light weights and do more reps. Work up a light sweat, not profusely perspiring. Don't push through the pain—pull back if you ache or feel a sharp pain. Even small movements will help synovial fluid flow into the achy area, lubricating dry joints and reducing inflammation. Always breathe through your nose when exercising, increasing nitrogen dioxide in the blood, which is healing. If you get out of breath, pull back until you can breathe through the nose again.

- Wear loose clothing to encourage blood flow to the area, but dress warmly. Light layers help to keep the lower back warm. Avoid exposing yourself to cold air and cold water.

- If you have access to a therapy pool or hot tub, soak often. Be sure that you can easily get in and out of the bath or pool, either on your own or with help. Remember to hydrate during and after your soak.

Panchakarma

If you are suffering from intense pain and cannot find relief, you may want to find a center where you can receive Panchakarma (Sanskrit for Five Actions). This 5,000-year-old treatment protocol uses various procedures to penetrate down to the cellular level to remove accumulated waste, ridding the body of debilitating toxins, and then slowly rejuvenating the body to a new level of wellness. Through diet, herbs, oils, steam, purgatives, enemas, nasal and eye washes, and deep rest, Panchakarma will address the entire body, allowing it to reset and regain function, elevating you at your absolute best.

It might seem like an indulgence to travel to a center to receive wholesome food, daily body massages, and encouragement to rest, but I have found this is simply the best way to address the stressors, environmental toxins, and immune-depleting activities of our daily lives. Ayurveda says that you cannot fix a machine while it is running. That means we need to stop, rest, and let someone else feed, oil, and heal us.

- Infrared and traditional saunas and steam rooms will help to ease lower back pain. Again, stay hydrated. Heating pads work well, too.

- Don't sit too long. Get up and move at least once an hour. Do leg lifts, either seated or holding on to the back of a chair or a table. Forward bends increase circulation to the lower back (page 36). Side bends and gentle twists will help, too. Nothing rigorous—all you need is 5 minutes of micro-movements several times a day to keep the blood moving.

- Maintain good posture. Walk around for a minute balancing a book on your head. Do balance poses such as tree pose. Feel your pelvic bones in neutral as you stand and sit tall, erect but not rigid.

APOTHECARY

- Try yogaraj guggulu and dashamula. These Ayurvedic herbs are traditional recommendations for back pain because they specifically help to balance Vata dosha and relieve pain. Take one to two tablets of yogaraj guggulu a day, before food. Dashamula is a combination of ten plant roots. Mix 1 tablespoon (15 g) in 4 to 6 ounces (120 to 175 ml) of hot water and let it sit for 5 to 10 minutes. Strain and drink. The rhizome Musta is another herb to try as it promotes healthy blood flow. Take ¼ to ½ teaspoon, two times a day, in 4 to 6 ounces (120 to 175 ml) of hot water. Do not use any of these remedies if pregnant.

- Apply any of the following oils to the area: mahanarayan, ashwagandha bala, nirgundi, and *karpooradi*. These amazing oils not only reduce pain but can actually heal injuries and lessen the progression of arthritis. Warm the oil of choice by placing the bottle in a glass of hot water or running it under hot water in the sink. Apply liberally to the area in pain. Do this three or four times a day, as needed. Keep it up every day even after the pain dissipates, as the mere act of applying and massaging oil to the skin keeps the tissues well lubricated and can prevent further injury.

- After applying oil, use a heating pad to keep the area warm and allow the oil to penetrate, for about 10 to 15 minutes. Place a towel or cloth that you won't mind getting oily between you and the heating pad.

Guided Meditation for Pain Relief

A relaxed mind and body can accomplish miraculous things, including reducing the amount of pain you feel. Meditation allows us to release the gripping, the holding, the tensing up that contribute to pain. Mind/body techniques help to loosen up and let go.

To use this meditation script for pain relief, read it and follow along with each step, closing your eyes and practicing each technique. Or record yourself, or have another person read it into a recorder and listen to it, pausing along the way until you feel you have mastered each step. Another way to integrate the meditation is simply to write it down yourself, copying it from this book into a journal.

See what resonates with you. Change or add a few things. For example, include a specific condition you are experiencing, or a time and place where you felt well. Make this healing meditation yours!

Find a place where you won't be distracted and sit comfortably. If you are in bed, try to raise your head with a few pillows so your body knows it's not time to sleep. Rather, it is time to meditate or contemplate.

Take a few deep breaths through your nose to the belly. Feel the air enter your nostrils and move to the back of your throat and down the windpipe, nourishing your body with each inhale and exhale. Breathe as deeply as possible.

Beginning with your toes, slowly scan your body. Notice how each segment feels. Wiggle, move, and stretch. There is no need to change anything you are feeling. Accept all in the moment, creating awareness. Noticing. Being fully present with what is.

Repeat silently to yourself:

I feel my toes. My big toes, I lift my big toes.
I lift my other toes. I notice how they feel.
I feel my foot. The arch, the sole, the heel.
I feel my ankles. Feeling my ankles connect to the calf and the lower leg.

Notice how this feels, and allow your attention to move up to your knees. Pause and repeat silently: *I feel my knees.* Go around your knees in your mind. Back and front and sides. Pay attention, offering gratitude for the work the knees perform, all the way down, connecting to your toes.

Reflect here and move up the thighs. Pause and repeat silently: *I feel my thighs, the fullness, the length, the femur bones that carry me around.* How is this all connected? What do you feel? Notice?

Moving from the thighs to the pelvis. Shifting a bit to find neutral. Pause and repeat silently: *I feel my hip bones. I see my pelvis, holding me in place.*

The pelvis bowl holds us and is most comfortable not too far back or too far forward. Shift in your seat and find that open space. Pause. Feel. Notice. Accept the feelings. Does movement improve pain one way or another? Find your space.

Let your attention flow to your lower back. Pause and notice your lower back and buttocks.

Is there discomfort here? Can you find the exact spot? Any place you feel pain, discomfort, or unease, pause and breathe into that space. Watch your breath and visualize it moving to that exact spot, expanding, and releasing.

Move around to your belly. Pause and repeat silently: *My soft belly. I let go.* Feel the expansion as you breathe into your belly. Place your hands on your stomach and breathe into your hands, feeling them rise on the inhale and lower on the exhale. Love your belly. Take three breaths here.

(continued)

Move to your chest, lungs, and ribs. Allow the breath to rise to this area. Feel the nourishment of the breath as it fills the torso and rib cage, as it fills the heart. Offering refreshment. Replenishment. Whole body healing. Pause and repeat silently: *I feel my ribs expand on the inhale. Filling me with life.*

Move your attention to your throat. Pause and ask yourself silently: *Do I speak my truth? Is there constriction? Is it open?* Hum. Feel the vibration awaken the vocal cords offering full-body healing as the hum moves up and down, to your toes and back up to your throat.

Hold the space for an opening as you move your attention to your neck, jaw, ears, cheeks, eyes, forehead. Loosening. Adjusting. Softening. Opening and closing the mouth. Feel your tongue move across your teeth and gums. Is there a sound you yearn to make out loud? Find that sound and emote, or allow yourself to be in silence.

Shift your attention to your entire head. Pause and repeat silently: *I feel my scalp.* Where is your mind? Allow it to be wherever it is, without pushing thoughts away. Accept. Recognize. Be present and aware.

Now that you have scanned your entire body, allow your focus to go where you noticed pain. Pinpoint the pain with laser focus. Don't shy away. Feel it. Recognize it. Compartmentalize it. Does it feel hot or cold? Dull or sharp? Pervasive or concentrated?

Spend some time here, applying your senses to the discomfort. Once you feel it's in your focus, give it a shape and a color. Visualize the area surrounding the pain. Is it red, blue, green, yellow? A square, circle, unformed?

Imagine you can breathe directly into the shape you have created. Breathe deeply. Watch the area expand and contract with each in breath and out breath. Where would you like it to go? Are you able to move the pain out of the body? Squeeze and contract it until it disintegrates into fine particles you can blow away.

THE BEGINNER'S GUIDE TO AYURVEDIC HOME REMEDIES

Visualize the fragments leaving your body. Maybe it will ease up or perhaps cease entirely. Let it go where it will. Remember you are in control at this moment. You decide how to handle the pain.

After you have worked with the pain area, allow your attention to flow where there is no pain. Spend time in those places and feel the absence of sensations. The space. The void. Remember what this feels like and when you feel the pain return, summon the void, the dispersed particles, and the space you have created.

Call to mind a time and place when you felt well. Whole. Fully healthy and happy. Where is that place?

What do you see? What is the weather like? Do you have a favorite food? What does it taste like? Are you with loved ones, a pet, or alone? What are you wearing? Are you walking or sitting? Relaxing? Reading? Watching a sunrise or sunset?

Bring this all to the front of your mind and watch yourself in that state of well-being. This is you. This is who you are and will always be. Rest in that space. Allow your thoughts to come and go without attempting to stop them or spend too much time on them, just flowing through the mind as you watch the show play out. Sit in this comfortable space for a few minutes. Relaxed. Renewed.

Slowly open your eyes and take in the wide world around you. Notice your part in the big picture. Take this feeling and perspective with you for the rest of your day. Whenever you feel the return of pain or discomfort, visualize the shape and color, and allow it to move on. See yourself as a whole, happy, pain-free being.

Practice this meditation as needed and you will begin to see your pain improve.

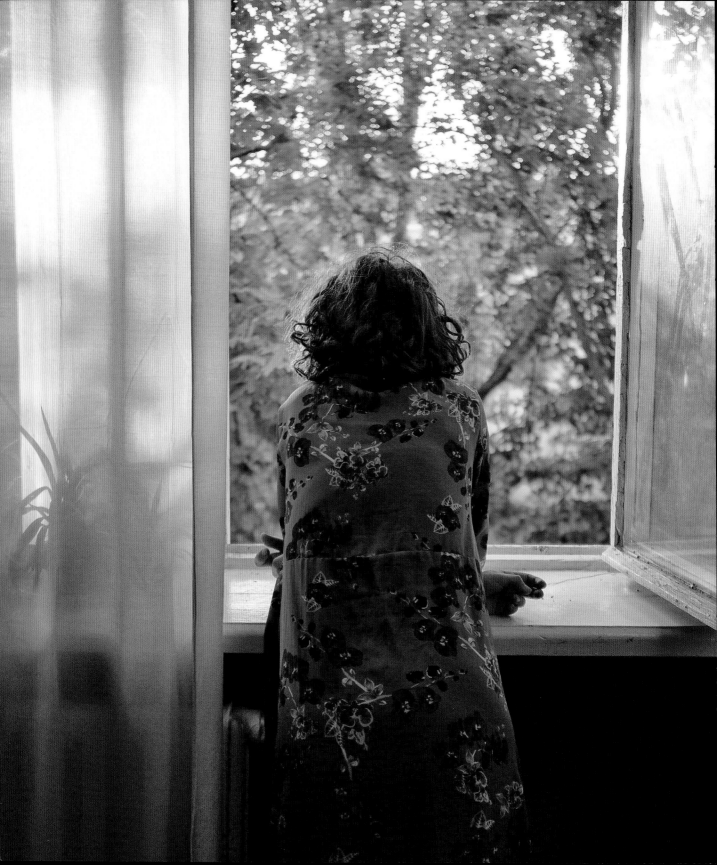

3

Respiratory System: Breathing into Perfect Health

Breath is life. In many languages the word for breath also means wind, soul, or spirit. We simply cannot live without breathing. We take a deep breath when we enter the world, and we exhale when we leave. It's actually quite elegant. While we are alive, how we use our breath can enhance our health or detract from it. In this chapter, we will learn how to utilize the breath in the most helpful ways, as well as how to heal when it is compromised.

Ayurveda, Breath, and Respiratory Ailments

"Just take a deep breath" or "Breathe and count to ten." We hear these sayings repeatedly when we are sad, crying, angry, or stressed out. It's natural to coach people to breathe as well as to soothe ourselves with deep breaths. Filling our lungs to capacity and slowly exhaling activates the parasympathetic nervous system, which is the opposite of "fight or flight." The parasympathetic creates a sense of calm and well-being, allowing us to relax, focus, and think, rather than lash out and react thoughtlessly. Think of the breath as a magic vapor that is available to us anytime. We must remember to use it.

The classical texts of Ayurveda, the *Charaka Samhita*, don't dwell too deeply on respiratory problems, perhaps because the air 5,000 years ago was not as contaminated as it is now. The text about breathing lyrically reads: "The *prana vayu* (air flow) traverses from the navel region through the throat, passes out to consume the nectar from the air in the atmosphere, and then comes back to nourish the body." If only that nectar still existed. Whether we live in a city, countryside, near the sea, on a mountaintop, or on a farm, chances are somewhere we will run into air contaminated with man-made or environmental toxins. If our immune system is compromised or we have become saturated with toxins, our lungs will suffer.

Ayurveda recognizes four types of respiratory ailments: rhinitis, sinusitis, breathing problems, and cough. Within each of these categories, the doshas express themselves differently.

- Vata will experience cough, colds, and lung ailments that produce a dry cough, lack of mucus, chest pain, laryngitis, and intermittent coughing fits.

- Pitta may be feverish, with a continuous cough, producing yellowish phlegm and a deeper infection.

- Kapha will have a constant cough, producing a whitish, sticky mucus, with a runny nose.

Ayurvedic Practices for Good Respiratory Health

As the doshas move across the lungs, Vata brings dryness, Pitta ignites inflammation, and Kapha saturates with phlegm. Food, supplements, and breath work mitigate the excess dosha to help the lungs open for easy airflow, without obstruction. To heal most effectively, avoid the cause of the irritation, nourish the tissues, and take preventative care.

FOOD: BREATHE EASY, EAT WHOLESOME

Eat omega-3 fatty acids and antioxidants. A diet that is rich in fish, nuts, seeds, and colorful fruits and vegetables is great for your respiratory system. Ayurveda also encourages us to eat whole foods, based on the season and any doshic imbalance you may have. Eat all the colors of the rainbow, for that season. Whatever the season and your doshic imbalance may be, white sugar, saturated fats, trans fats, and processed foods create a host of symptoms; avoid them at all times, especially if you are having sinus or breathing problems.

Eat seasonally. Food that is available in season will protect you from many ailments. Pay attention to what is traditionally available either at your local farmers' market or in your own garden, and begin to cultivate knowledge of seasonal eating.

Consume warm food when it's cold and room temperature/cool food when it's hot. It can really be that simple! Avoid iced-cold drinks on a snowy day. Choose chilled tea over hot cocoa in summer. Ayurveda suggests staying away from very cold as it puts out our digestive fires, but a cool drink on a hot day can be very soothing. Just don't go crazy with the ice! Eating and drinking with the season, rather than against it, allows the body to maintain its natural, seasonal microbiome, which builds immunity, strengthens the tissues, and promotes good digestive health, feeding the mind and spirit as well.

LIFESTYLE: PROTECT AND NOURISH THE RESPIRATORY SYSTEM

Practice breath work. Getting in the habit of doing breath work before you are sick boosts lung capacity and builds immunity. Any deep breath work like alternate nostril breathing, boxed breathing, or sheetali (see pages 174, 175, and 177) will help to keep the lungs clear, allowing you to pull air deep into the pockets of the lungs, and fully expel the breath, ridding the body of toxins. (If you are sick, do what you can, but don't overdo it. Allow yourself time to rest, but keep breathing in gently, out of the deepest recesses of the lungs.)

Make wise purchases to benefit your health. Many conventional detergents leave a layer of chemicals on your clothes to repel stains and dirt, and prevent wrinkling. You really don't want those chemicals next to your skin all day or in your sheets and towels. Wear clean, organic fibers and wash clothes in natural detergents, such as soap nuts or one of the many natural products on the market.

Do not use traditional fabric softeners. They are extremely toxic and leave a chemical residue on your clothes, sheets, and towels. Use natural, plant-based dryer sheets or balls or other natural products. Read the ingredients and if it is not plant-based, don't use it.

Avoid adding chemicals to your home. This includes room and furniture sprays and other chemical-laden products that mask odors, including plug-ins and diffusers. These are major irritants to the lungs of not only you, but your pets as well. They contain known cancer-causing chemicals.

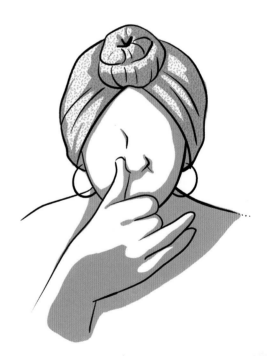

If you live in a polluted area, wear a mask like a KN-95 or N-95 when outdoors. We've all become accustomed to these masks during COVID-19, but people in places such as Delhi, Bombay, and Hong Kong have been wearing masks outdoors for years as their air quality has deteriorated. They are effective for prevention.

Wear clothing appropriate to the climate. Wearing a scarf anytime it's windy or there is a touch of a chill in the air can make you less vulnerable to getting sick. Wear layers that trap warmth against your body, which can also be easily discarded when the temperature changes. Yes, it's true that germs cause disease, but our body can weaken when it needs to rev up its energy for basics like staying warm, when that energy can be used toward other important immune functions like metabolizing food and detoxification.

APOTHECARY: BREATHE EASY BEFORE YOU HAVE AN ISSUE

Quercetin. There are so many reasons to take quercetin regularly. It is great for allergies (page 81). Studies show that it may suppress cancer growth and protect against degenerative brain disorders like dementia and Alzheimer's. To sing quercetin's praises even more, recent research shows that this plant pigment flavonoid may even help prevent COVID-19 and other coronaviruses. Experts say that quercetin lowers blood pressure, increases longevity, and controls blood sugar.

Sesame seed oil. Gargle with it every day. After you brush your teeth, take a tablespoon of sesame seed oil and gargle for about 20 to 30 seconds and spit into a trash can. This is called *kavala* in Sanskrit.

Closely related to this practice is *gandusha*, or oil pulling, which is another beneficial daily practice. For gandusha, take 1 tablespoon (15 ml) of sesame seed or coconut oil in the mouth and slowly swish, hold for 15 minutes, and spit into a trash can. Both practices are antibacterial and antifungal and create a protective barrier from toxins in the mouth. Gandusha and kavala can protect from bacterial invaders in the body and reduce inflammation.

Condition: Cough, Colds, Sore Throat, Non-Asthmatic Breathing Problems

Environmental conditions, infections, and even overuse of the voice from talking too much, singing, or shouting can cause irritation of the throat, resulting in a cough, a scratchy throat, or breathing difficulties. Beyond rest and recuperation, think about warm, soothing food and drink to heal and reduce symptoms. If we think back to what our grandmothers or a wise elder would advise, it's usually the way to go: hot water with lemon and honey; ginger tea; chicken soup or a version thereof; and Vicks VapoRub.

There are Ayurvedic versions for these, including the tried-and-true honey, ginger, lemon concoctions, and eucalyptus oils.

In terms of prevention, always wear a scarf around the throat when the weather cools down. I even wear one around the house. Keep a thermos of warm water with you when you are outside your home so that you can sip and stay hydrated throughout the day. Take a break from talking so much and try listening more. It is better for your throat, and you will probably learn something new. Try to avoid smoke-filled areas. Seek fresh air as often as you can.

FOOD

- As with most things in Ayurveda, healing begins in the gut. All doshas should avoid excessive dairy and lean toward bitter, heating, and astringent foods such as bitter leafy greens, cilantro, parsley, lemons, limes, raw honey, and ginger.

- Avoid ice, cold, and raw food. Eat soups, stews, rice, or quinoa bowls with greens and protein.

Soothing Teas

Ginger, *tulsi*, or turmeric tea (with raw honey and lemon) will soothe the throat and reduce the inflammatory response for all three doshas. Sip as a hot tea throughout the day or buy throat lozenges made from these products.

Drink licorice tea if you have a lot of mucus and coughing. A hot cup of licorice tea can help soothe a hard cough and open up your breathing. Use ¼ to ½ teaspoon licorice powder in 10 to 12 ounces (285 to 355 ml) hot water. Sip 1 to 2 cups a day. Do not use if you are pregnant.

Green tea contains many beneficial nutrients, including a natural histamine that counters allergies. Enjoy 1 or 2 cups a day to help you through allergy season. Be aware, though, that tea is dehydrating so be sure to have a glass of water after your tea.

LIFESTYLE

- Do not smoke, vape, or be around people who are smoking.

- Do yoga poses that open the chest, ribs, and lungs such as cobra, bridge, camel, and chest openers, such as lying on a bolster.

- Breathe in fresh air as much as possible. If you are sick in bed, keep a window open to allow fresh, clean air to circulate, or use a HEPA (high-efficiency particulate air) filter to purify the air.

APOTHECARY

- *Sitopaladi* is an herb blend used for an unproductive cough, or a cough with white or yellow phlegm. It's a tasty mixture of sugar, cinnamon, cardamom, pippali, and bamboo sap, and it is one of the most popular Ayurvedic remedies. It is widely available online and in Indian food stores. Take in powder form, 1 to 2 tablespoons (5 to 10 ml) either mixed into a paste with a bit of hot water and licked off a spoon, or made into a tea with 10 to 12 ounces (285 to 355 ml) of hot water. Take it once or twice a day. There are no contraindications.

Breathe Free Soup

This recipe combines herbs and spices to clarify the lungs and open the airways. It's perfect for seasonal allergy time and for treating coughs and colds.

Makes 4 servings

- ½ red onion, chopped
- 3 cloves garlic, minced
- 1 tablespoon (15 ml) extra-virgin olive oil or ghee
- 1–2 tablespoons (7–13 g) chopped fresh ginger
- 2 dried red chiles (optional)
- 1 teaspoon red pepper flakes
- 1 teaspoon *ajwain*
- 1 teaspoon ground turmeric
- 1 teaspoon sea salt
- 1 teaspoon black pepper
- ½ teaspoon ground cardamom
- Pinch of ground cloves
- 6 cups (1.4 L) veggie stock or water
- 1 carrot, diced
- 1 stalk celery, chopped
- 1 (6-inch or 15-cm) daikon radish, chopped
- 1–2 teaspoons (5–10 ml) hot sauce (If you are Pitta dosha, go for less)
- 2 tablespoons (28 ml) tamari
- Juice of 1 lime
- 1 cup (235 ml) canned, full-fat coconut milk

Sauté the onion and garlic in olive oil or ghee in a large soup pot over medium heat for 3 minutes, until softened. Be careful not to burn the garlic. Stir in the spices and cook for 30 seconds, or until aromatic.

Add the stock and stir in the veggies and hot sauce. Bring to a boil, then reduce the heat and simmer for 20 minutes.

Stir in the coconut milk and simmer for 5 minutes. Blend in the pot with an immersion blender if you want a smooth soup, or let it cool a bit and carefully add to a blender. Add tamari and lime juice to taste before serving. Enjoy the soup in a bowl or sip it from a mug.

NOTES

- Play around with the amount of spices to find the best flavor and healing elixir for you. Don't be afraid to try new herbs and spices in various combinations as they are all medicinal.

- If you're not feeling well and soup feels like too much heat, add more water or broth to thin it out for more of an elixir.

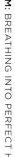

- The ingredients in *talisadi* are the same as those in sitopaladi, with the addition of ginger, pepper, and *talisa*. Use this formula if you have a wet cough to break up mucus. Talisadi aids upset stomachs, fever, diarrhea, or indigestion. Take 1 to 2 tablespoons (15 to 30 g) as a paste or in a tea, once or twice a day.

- If you have a sore throat, gargle two to three times a day with warm water, ½ teaspoon salt, and ½ teaspoon turmeric powder. Additionally, gargle with coconut oil or sesame oil. Take 1 tablespoon (15 ml), gargle three or four times, and spit the oil into a trash can to avoid clogging pipes.

Ajwain

Also known as carom seeds, ajwain is considered antiseptic. It is a great remedy for stomach ailments, digestive problems, colds, and headache. Soak 1 tablespoon (15 g) in 12 ounces (355 ml) of hot water for 30 minutes (or overnight), strain, and drink.

- Rub the chest with a balm containing eucalyptus, camphor, clove, and menthol. Banyan Botanicals makes an effective product called *Breathe Free* with these and other supporting herbs, which you can apply to the chest, back, and under the nose. You may also mix those essential oils, just two to three drops each, with 2 ounces (60 ml) of a carrier oil like sesame or jojoba and apply as directed.

- Rest in a warm bath of Epsom salts and a few drops of lung-clearing essential oils, such as eucalyptus or peppermint. Place a warm washcloth over your chest while in the bath. If you don't have a bathtub, put ten drops of eucalyptus oil around the edges of your shower and take a hot shower.

- Always dress appropriately and wear a neck scarf if it is cool or windy outside. Wear layers to adjust your body temperature to the cold, and it's better to stay bundled up if you are suffering from a lung ailment.

Essential Oil Steam

To break up mucus and help the lungs heal, try an essential oil steam: Add three drops each of lavender, eucalyptus, and tea tree oil to a large bowl of steaming hot water. Drape a towel over your head, find a comfortable distance from the bowl, close your eyes, and inhale and exhale deeply for five to ten breaths. Do this two to three times a day. These oils will help to open the passageways of the bronchial tubes, reduce inflammation, and kill bacterial infections.

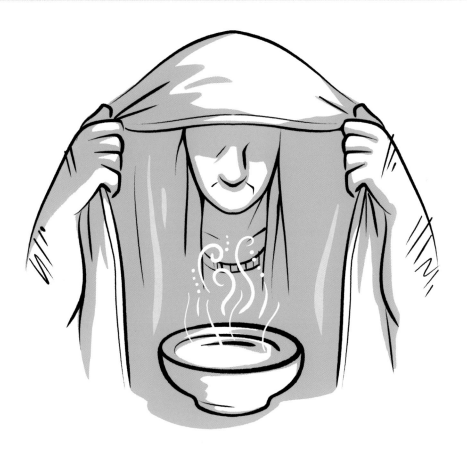

Condition: Sinusitis

Sinusitis symptoms include facial pain, stuffed and inflamed nasal passages, headache, and pain in the neck and jaw.

Follow all the guidelines for a cough, cold, and sore throat with these additional tips:

- Use a neti pot (page 78) solution of ¼ teaspoon salt and a pinch of baking soda. Rinse your nasal passages once or twice a day.

- Consider adding Neti Wash from Himalayan Chandra to your neti pot water. It contains eucalyptus, peppermint, and menthol. They also have a wash with zinc that may be useful.

- Place a very warm washcloth with a drop or two of eucalyptus or peppermint essential oil on your face. Press deeply into your sinus areas, avoiding the eyes.

If the problem persists for more than five days, you may need medical intervention and antibiotics. Continue the above protocols even if you need to take antibiotics, Just add in a probiotic. Take one probiotic capsule a day while on the antibiotic and continue for thirty days.

Condition: Rhinitis

Rhinitis is a disorder of too much water, exacerbated by toxins. The condition differs from sinusitis as the inflamed tissues are in the mucus membranes of the nose (as opposed to the sinuses). If you are suffering from rhinitis, you may have a runny nose, a scratchy or itchy throat, and watery eyes. This reaction is often caused by environmental toxins such as perfumes, mold, mildew, dust, smoke, animal dander, and even waste from insects and rodents.

When you have a general feeling of aches or pains, or sinus, nasal, or throat issues, and they have no pathological roots, it is a clear indication that something is wrong in the environment. When I work with clients who feel unwell much of the time, I ask them to search their home for the root cause. If you are feeling attacked with symptoms, see if there are any obvious causes in your environment. If you have recently moved to a new home, check for mold. If you live in a cluttered space, clean it up and throw out items damaged by water or infestation. Remove all possible toxins from your environment.

If gone untreated, rhinitis may lead to nasal polyps and even asthma. Rid yourself of these symptoms by following all the protocols for respiratory health (page 67) and don't close the door on a cluttered space or push dust under the rug or bed. We must have a clean home, free of toxins, to maintain our health. A lotus may be able to grow in the mud, but we can't function well in a house filled with clutter, chemicals, and hidden waste. Clean up as best you can.

Try Quercetin for Rhinitis

Rhinitis is a histamine response to allergens. An antihistamine supplement, like quercetin, helps to heal allergic reactions through antioxidant and anti-inflammatory actions. Many studies indicate this plant supplement may prevent certain cancers, heart disease, and inflammatory issues. For more on quercetin, see page 85.

To treat rhinitis: Take two capsules once a day with food until your symptoms cease.

To treat acute cases: Take two tablets twice a day, for seven days. Do not take if you are pregnant, are breastfeeding, or have kidney issues.

When and How to Use a Neti Pot

A neti pot is a form of nasal irrigation and helps to remove excess mucus, debris, allergens, and toxins from the nasal passages. It reduces inflammation and irritation, and helps to detoxify the entire body. The nose is our first line of defense to the environment, so when we clean it out and oil the tissues, we are providing a clean canvas to catch toxins and prevent them from entering the body and causing disturbances. Many people use their neti pots for seasonal allergies, or when they have been in a polluted atmosphere.

Neti pots are widely available online, in health food and grocery stores, and at pharmacies. Choose one that is ceramic for home and one made of unbreakable material, such as recycled plastic, for travel to use after being on an airplane or in a polluted city.

- Neti pot
- Boiling water to fill the pot, cooled to warm
- Pharmaceutical-grade salt made for neti pots
  (Or use a salt that is *not* iodized.)
- Tissues
- Towel
- Nasya oil, sesame oil, or ghee

Fill the pot with boiled water that has cooled. Stir in ¼ teaspoon of neti pot salt. DO NOT use iodized salt in your neti pot.

Lean over a sink and tilt your head to the side, with your ear over your shoulder and chin slightly tucked. Place the tip of the pot in your upper nostril and begin to slowly pour the water into your nasal passage. Breathe evenly though your mouth. The water should pour out the lower nostril into the sink.

Continue until the pot is empty. If you feel water in your ear or throat, adjust your head and the tilt of your chin until the water is just running out of your nose.

Have a tissue handy and blow gently to clear excess water. Refill the pot with your saltwater mixture. Tilt your head to the other side and repeat.

When you are done, gently blow your nose. Bend at the waist and lean forward, letting your head hang for a few seconds.

To assist with draining your nose, you can do windmills by touching your left toes with your right hand and reaching up toward the ceiling with the left arm. Turn your head to the side to look at the upturned arm. Repeat on the opposite side. Hold on each side for about 10 seconds.

Wait at least one hour for the nasal passages to dry, then apply nasya oil, sesame seed oil, or ghee. Just place a few drops on your pinky and swirl around the inside of your nose, coating the tissues and gently coating the sinuses.

If you live in a dry climate, skip the neti pot and just use nasya oil several times a day as needed. Take nasya oil with you when you travel, as hotels and airplanes are drying.

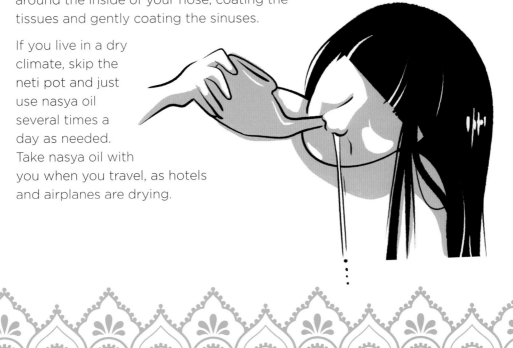

FOOD

- If you are experiencing a runny nose and watery eyes, avoid all dairy and heavy, wet, cold food. That means no yogurt, cheese, milk, butter, or fast or fried food. Avoid white sugar. Notice how you feel after eating wheat, such as pasta or bread. If you see an increase in symptoms, avoid it.

- Follow a Kapha-reducing plan of less dairy, sugar, and wheat. Add in some spicy foods to heat up the excess mucus, such as green chiles, a dash of cayenne pepper, and premixed hot curry powder. Add these to rice, soups, stews, and veggies.

- Eat leafy greens and vegetables, especially bitter ones, such as dandelion greens, mustard greens, radicchio, daikon radish, cilantro, and parsley.

- Make licorice or green tea (page 71) to sip throughout the day. (Avoid licorice if you are pregnant.)

LIFESTYLE

- Clean up your house. Remove anything that might be an allergen, such as perfumes or scented cleaners, sprays, dishwashing liquid, and detergents. Even soap and shampoo may be what is causing you trouble.

- Use an air filter to purify the air.

- If you have a pet, notice if your eyes get watery or your nose runs while the pet is around. If so, you may need to keep the pet off your furniture and the bed and vacuum regularly. Homeopathic pet dander remedies are effective as well. (I would never tell you to get rid of your pet!)

- Open doors and windows unless it is high pollen season. Allowing fresh air to circulate will bring in more oxygen, enabling our bodies to better battle the toxins.

- On hot, humid days, run your air conditioner at 74°F (23°C) or less to keep the air pure and less humid. On rainy or humid days, use a dehumidifier to dry out the air. Less moist air is better for your health in this situation.

- Wash all towels, sheets, blankets, and clothes in nontoxic detergents. If your fabrics are contaminated with dander or mildew or are otherwise stained, try a wash with borax powder. If that does not work, buy new ones, beginning with one set of organic sheets or a new towel. Slowly replace your linens and clothes until you are allergen-free.

APOTHECARY

- Use a neti pot with saline water and a pinch of turmeric. This will reduce the inflamed tissues in the nose. If your nose is too stuffed, try pouring the water in anyway and allow it to run out the same nostril. The turmeric/salt mix will still have some effect.

- Do the essential oil steam (page 75) with three drops each of lavender, eucalyptus, and tea tree oil in a large bowl of steaming hot water. Drape a towel over your head, find a comfortable distance from the bowl, close your eyes, and inhale and exhale deeply for five to ten breaths. Do this two to three times a day.

- Gargle with warm water with ½ teaspoon of salt and ½ teaspoon of turmeric, three to four times a day.

Condition: Seasonal Conditions and Allergies

Each season brings on its own set of issues. Winter brings dry noses and throats, while spring and summer bring runny eyes, sneezing, congestion, and excess mucus. Ayurveda recommends we practice the opposite attributes of the season. When it's cold and damp outside, eat warm and dry food. When it's hot and dry out, eat cool and moist food. Hot and humid? Go for cool and dry. In variable climates, stick to simple, seasonal foods that are easy to digest. All of this will combat seasonal allergies and conditions as they arise.

FOOD

- Fall and winter are considered dry and cold. This brings on constipation as well as dry sinuses and scratchy, sore throats.

  To remedy: Concentrate on foods that are warm, hearty, and heavy. Think stews, soups, and some meat. Organic dairy, such as plain yogurt, butter, cream, and milk (goat or cow), is more effectively digested in winter, as our digestive fires are higher and easily break down these heavier foods. Whole grains and complex carbohydrates such as brown rice, oatmeal, potatoes, beans, peas, and lentils are included in these heavier foods and prevent winter ailments such as cough and cold by feeding the gut what it needs.

- Springtime is considered cool, damp, and variable. Greens and flowers bloom, rains fall, roots shoot up, and plant and tree pollen fill the air. These environmental changes cause some people to suffer from allergies. Watery eyes, excess mucus in the nose, phlegm in the lungs, and even hives and rashes from undetermined causes are just some common allergic reactions.

  To remedy: Nature offers so many remedies in spring. Look for spring growth of asparagus, ramps, green beans, radishes, spinach, leafy greens, rhubarb, peas, and artichokes. All of these foods are nature's remedies to detox from heavy winter intake. Cilantro and parsley help to detox the heaviness of winter foods. Raw honey will scrape out excess water and dampness and provide nutrients that will please the gut. It's important to use only raw honey as pasteurized honey is heated to such high levels that it kills off the propolis, nutrients, minerals, and enzymes that make honey such an amazing superfood. Certain fruits, such as apples and pears, help to dry up mucus as well.

- Summer is hot, and it's humid or dry. Excessive heat and sun cause sunstroke, dehydration, sunburn, headaches, and fatigue.

Nasya Oil

The dry season irritates the mucosal lining of the nose, and the nose is our first line of defense against allergies and respiratory issues. It's important to keep those tissues lubricated to help the immune system ward off bacteria.

Apply nasya oil regularly to keep the nose primed and ready to block invaders. Nasya oil comes with a dropper to apply the oil. Just place three to five drops directly into the nose and squeeze the nostrils together while taking a quick nasal inhale to absorb and disperse the oil. You may also put some drops on your pinky and swirl the oil in the nostrils. Use the oil any time you feel you need it.

To remedy: Watermelon, honeydew, and cantaloupe will hydrate the tissues just as efficiently as drinking a glass of water. Other hydrating, watery foods include coconuts, zucchinis, peaches, mangoes, and plums. Reduce caffeine, which increases blood flow to the skin, creating heat. Ghee is cooling and sweet, which is the perfect antidote to the heat. Adding freshly ground chia or flaxseeds to soups, smoothies, or cereals will quench thirst as they are gelatinous and provide moisture.

LIFESTYLE

- **Fall and Winter.** Warm, fall days lead to cool nights, so wear layers. Always wear a scarf to protect your throat from wind and cold.

  In the chill of winter, indoor spaces may be overheated. Use a humidifier in your home if it's dry. This will help keep nasal passages and your throat lubricated, which allows more efficient protection from toxins.

- **Spring.** Spring brings heavy rains, which lead to warm, humid evenings and cool mornings. Whenever the weather is changing throughout the day, having light layers, like a scarf, is important. Always protect the neck and throat.

  On high pollen days consider wearing a mask outdoors. Inside, keep air circulating with fans or use your heat/air system on circulation mode or an air-purifying filtration system. If you live in a high pollen area, it's best to keep the windows closed, but after a clearing rain, open them wide for the fresh air.

  Spring is an ideal time to use a neti pot (see page 78). Use the pot once in the morning with a saline wash. Allow the nostrils to dry fully for one hour, then apply nasya oil, ghee, or sesame seed oil to the tissues inside the nasal passages.

- **Summer.** Allergens cause havoc in summer because we tend to spend more time outside. Grass, trees, ragweed, moldy leaves, and freshly cut grass all cause allergic reactions in some people. When you are outdoors, consider wearing a mask covering your mouth and nose.

  Hot, warm air traps the allergens in the atmosphere and even in your house, where mold, mildew, and dust mites proliferate. To prevent indoor allergens, keep the humidity low, between 30 to 50 percent, by running a dehumidifier. Run the air conditioner and keep the windows closed. Vacuum often and use a filtration machine. Keep dust at bay by using unscented microfiber dusters.

Be Free of Allergies Smoothie

This smoothie is packed with flavonoids, phytonutrients, and vitamin C. The bee pollen and raw honey provide enzymes, propolis, vitamins, and minerals. It packs a punch to help your system get rid of spring and summer allergens and irritations. Drink this if you are affected by seasonal allergies, or as a boost to the immune system. Take on an empty stomach and don't eat again until you feel hungry. If you leave the peel on the orange, it adds extra allergy-busting flavonoids and an exciting bitter bite to the drink! If it is your first time using bee pollen, use ½ teaspoon for the first week, then gradually add more.

Makes 2 servings

- 1½ cups (355 ml) boxed (not canned) shelf-stable coconut milk or any nondairy milk
- ½ cup (120 ml) warm water, plus more if needed
- 1 tablespoon (20 g) raw, organic honey (local if possible)
- ½–1 tablespoon (8–15 g) bee pollen
- 1 tablespoon (15 ml) flaxseed oil
- 1 unpeeled apple, cored and chopped
- 1 orange, chopped or sliced
- ½ cup (75 g) fresh or frozen blueberries
- 1-inch (2.5 cm) fresh ginger, peeled
- 1 teaspoon turmeric powder
- 1 cup (30 g) fresh spinach

Add the coconut milk, water, honey, bee pollen, and oil to a blender, then add the fruit, ginger, turmeric, and spinach. Whir it up until liquefied. Add more warm water if needed. Drink right away or, if you need to store it in the fridge, pour into an airtight glass jar. It will be good for 24 hours. Bring back to room temp or add hot water to warm it up if cold, before drinking.

APOTHECARY

- The allergy regimen I most often prescribe to my clients is a mix of Western and Eastern medicine. It seems to work well for all doshas in all seasons. If you are having allergic reactions, try this:

  » Take quercetin. This flavonoid acts as an antioxidant with amazing powers to combat inflammation and allergy symptoms. It is found in grapes, cherries, berries, apples, onions, and even green tea, coffee, and red wine. Taking it as a supplement offers the boost needed during allergy season. I usually suggest two capsules once or twice a day (500 to 1,000 mg a day). You may take the same amount during the rest of the year for all the other benefits it offers. Taking quercetin with vitamin C boosts the benefits, and many brands contain both. There are no negative side effects or contraindications.

  » In my personal experience, quercetin doesn't just block allergy symptoms, it heals, allowing you to use the supplement for three to six months (if you just want to take for allergy relief), and that's it! It adjusts the body to stop reacting to allergens. Most of my clients report a cessation of symptoms. If your allergies do return, take the capsules for a few weeks during the highest irritation periods to boost the system and prevent further irritation.

  » Try Pollen Protect from Banyan Botanicals. This Ayurvedic remedy is a formulation of ten key herbs for suppressing the allergic response, reducing inflammation and mucus. I haven't found a better Ayurvedic product. At the onset of the season, take two tablets twice a day after food. During acute phases, take three tablets three times a day. Always take it with about 10 ounces (285 ml) of water. If you are nursing, consult a practitioner before taking. Pollen Protect and quercetin plus vitamin C can be taken together.

- I do not recommend using antihistamines. Antihistamines or antihistamine sprays dry out the system and do not address the root cause of the allergens. Drying the mucosal lining will stop sneezing and nose blowing, but ultimately leads to far more damage as your natural ability to block toxins is removed. We need to have moist, lubricated nasal passages. Using oil and other supplements and following these steps will soothe the nasal passages rather than irritating and drying them with conventional formulas.

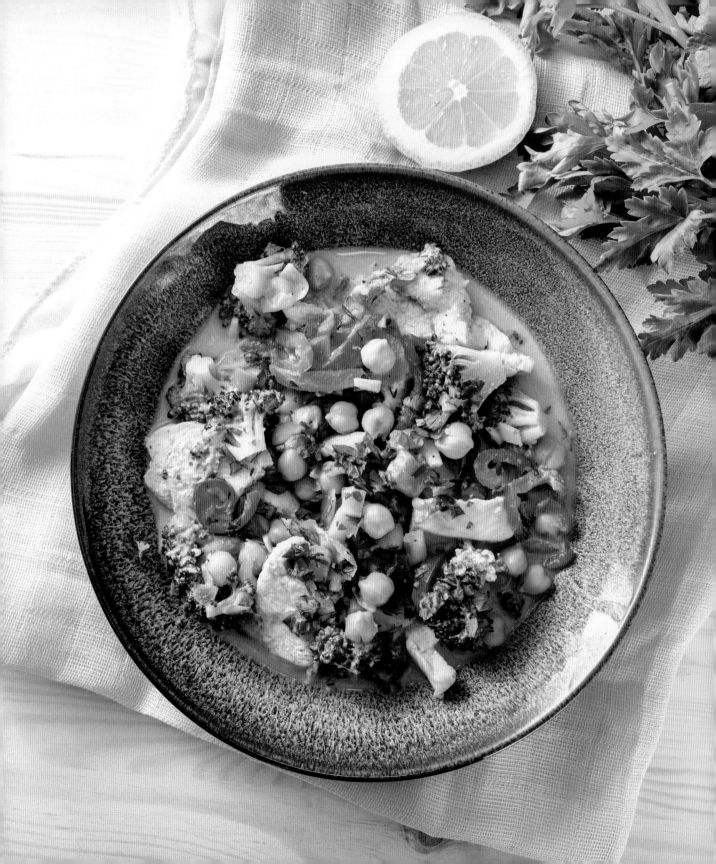

4

Digestion: Mouth, Gut, Assimilation, and Elimination

Food nourishes our mind, body, and spirit—that is brain, physical body, and your mood. In Ayurveda, fire—or *agni*—is one of the elements that makes up the doshas. When we talk about digestion, it is the fire in the belly that metabolizes our food, thoughts, desires, needs, and wants, creating a link between what we eat, how we feel, and what we think. The methods discussed here keep agni at optimal levels.

Ayurveda and Good Digestive Health

Modern science has identified serotonin, oxytocin, and dopamine as our happy hormones. They are produced in the gut and affect the brain. The vagus nerve makes the actual physical connection between the gut and the brain. It is a tentacle-like nerve that begins at the brain stem, branches out, and winds through the torso to the base of the spine, hugging our organs along the way. It is one of twelve cranial nerves whose effect on us is so vast that it has been called the body's information highway.

Nutritional psychiatry is taking a deep look at how food affects the hormones we secrete, and our mental and physical health. The vagus nerve stimulates the parasympathetic nervous system, which, unlike the sympathetic nervous system (which controls our fight-or-flight response), makes us feel safe, calm, and well. The vagus nerve helps us to rest and digest. When healthy, it signals the digestive tract and muscles in our stomach to push food through, by contracting and moving it to the small intestine. What we eat directly affects our mood, emotions, and brain. When you don't eat well, you and the digestive tract are unhappy.

In Ayurveda, the gut-brain connection is fueled by a healthy agni (fire) and the strength of the vagus nerve. Agni must be stoked and primed to be most effective. Studies have established that conditions such as anxiety, depression, and other emotional disorders are directly related to food choices. We know this is true for physical diseases, such as diabetes, heart disease, and some cancers. Now, the link is being made between what you eat, when you eat it, and how you feel.

Digestion is paramount to good health. Food, thoughts, images, sensations, and feelings all need to be digested properly for us to be healthy. The quality of each of these is what makes up our entire being. If we are constantly eating fast food, watching violent movies, or living in a cluttered, dank, dark environment, that will all be reflected in our physical and mental health.

With that in mind, consuming whole food in a space that is pleasing is the ultimate healthy eating practice. Sit down, be mindful and grateful, and pay attention to each bite. Vata can forget to eat or rush through meals. Pitta gets so hungry that they can wolf down a meal in minutes. Kapha loves to linger and may end up eating too much. Try to find your own balance. An enjoyable meal is more likely to be digested more efficiently.

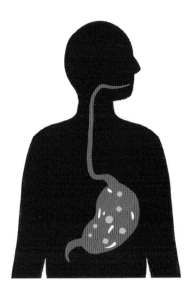

FOOD

- Eat a variety of healthy, seasonal foods. Our guts adjust by constantly sorting through good and bad bacteria, feeding most happily on the naturally occurring flora and fauna of the season. This feeds the gut microbiome as it shifts with the time of year. These good bacteria in the gut help break down food into useful components that keep the lining of the stomach and intestines healthy, supporting the process that creates a healthy mind and body. Boost the microbiome by choosing both prebiotic and probiotic foods, which benefit mental as well as physical health.

Probiotic and Prebiotic Foods

All the following will bolster your digestion by feeding the gut microbiome exactly what it needs to function at the highest level. If you do not already eat these foods, introduce them slowly into your diet and see how you feel. Increase your intake until they are a regular part of your everyday routine.

Probiotic Foods
- Unsweetened, full-fat yogurt and *kefir* from grass-fed cows or goats
- Fermented vegetables, such as sauerkraut or kimchi
- Tempeh (fermented soybeans)
- Miso paste (added to soups, rice, etc.)
- Kombucha
- Pickles

Prebiotic Foods
- Dandelion greens (just like the ones that grow in your yard; without pesticides or herbicides)
- Berries
- Bananas
- Garlic, leeks, and onions
- Asparagus
- Chickpeas, legumes, and lentils

- Take care of your digestive system. There are many more probiotic and prebiotic foods to choose from, so investigate and incorporate. But eating well is only half of it. You must be able to absorb the nutrients deep into the tissues, bones, and blood. We love to say, "You aren't what you eat. You are what you absorb, digest, and assimilate." As you metabolize the nutrients, toxins move out of the body through bowel movements, urine, sweat, and menstrual blood. Food assimilated and waste eliminated.

- Healthy digestion depends on all the links of the system working together. Prevent health problems and keep your body strong by choosing organic, fresh, seasonal, and varied foods. Use good oils. Eat high-fiber, low-sugar foods. Enjoy easy-to-digest proteins, nuts and seeds, fresh fruits, greens, and vegetables. If you eat meat, choose organic, humanely raised. And if you eat fish, choose wild caught (never farmed as it's less nutritious, and, frankly, horrible for the fish).

- Avoid all processed foods. These contain chemicals and preservatives, food coloring, and a variety of harmful additives. A good rule to follow is if the food is packaged and has more than seven ingredients, put it back on the shelf. If you consistently eat with these guidelines in place, you'll avoid many issues that affect the gastrointestinal system. Your bowel movements will be well formed and consistent. Stomachaches will resolve themselves, heartburn will disappear, and your weight will stabilize.

LIFESTYLE

- Take a walk after your meals for at least 10 minutes. To promote healthy digestion, get regular exercise—20 to 30 minutes three or four times a week at least. It's important to choose something you like (you'll be more likely to stick with it) and be sure to pace yourself, especially if you've been sedentary for a while. It can be tempting to overexert before your body is ready for it. Ayurveda suggests not overtaxing yourself in this way. Movement after meals keeps the blood flowing, which promotes digestion, rather than stagnation.

- Reduce your stress by reducing stressful situations. Easier said than done, but make a proactive effort. Only watch as much news as you need to be informed. Don't watch scary or violent movies or TV shows. Read books that are uplifting or helpful. Listen to calming music. Look at beautiful images. Turn off the computer or tablet at least an hour before bed and snuggle up to a loved one or a pet, or write in a gratitude journal.

- Good digestion also relies on healthy sleep patterns. That means being in bed by 10 p.m., which is Pitta time of night. During the hours of 10 p.m. until 2 a.m., your digestive system revs up and metabolizes everything you took in during the day. For this process to be completed, it is best to have a light dinner, putting less stress on the body to extract nutrients and prepare waste for elimination.

APOTHECARY

- *Triphala*. This is a combination of three Indian fruits that, together, act as a bowel toner and cleanser. Most people do well taking two tablets with warm water before bed. Triphala can regulate constipation and loose stools, and maintain healthy bowel movements. It's helpful to work with a practitioner to get the right dosage for your situation.

- Warm water. Drinking 12 to 16 ounces (355 to 475 ml) of warm water in the morning, after your oral care, gets the digestive juices churning. You can add a squeeze of lemon or a half teaspoon of apple cider vinegar if you'd like, or just drink it straight.

Rejoice in Who You Truly Are!

The gut microbiome plays a key role in all digestive and mental health. Your takeaway here is to eat a wide variety of fresh, whole foods, avoid overeating and night eating, and introduce probiotic and prebiotic foods into your meals every day. Stay hydrated, avoid alcohol and sugars, and eat food that is easy on the tummy.

I promise, if you do all this *and* reduce stress in your life through proper sleep, meditation, and movement, many if not all your digestive issues will disappear. Your weight will stabilize at the right number for you and your dosha. Ignore the BMI. Look at the dosha to understand your natural-born body type (page 11).

Teeth and Oral Care

So much of Ayurvedic wellness is about the digestive process. That process begins way before you put the food in your mouth. It actually starts when you think about food: what you are craving, how it will be prepared, and when it will be consumed. Saliva forms long before food is in the mouth and protects your teeth from the assaulting foods. It contains chemicals that neutralize acids, protecting enamel and fighting off tooth decay.

That is just one reason why oral care is paramount to good health. Tooth decay may affect the heart and other organs. Be vigilant about oral hygiene and care for your gums, teeth, and tongue. Like the gut, the mouth is teeming with good and bad bacteria called the oral microbiome. When you are healthy, saliva produces bacteria that will protect your enamel and increase digestibility. Eating too many sugary, sticky, gummy-like foods harms your teeth and impedes digestion. This includes soda, hard candy, milkshakes, coffee drinks, alcohol, and even dried fruit.

The best way to begin your day is to wash your mouth the Ayurvedic way, before you eat or drink anything. As the metabolism digests food during the night, bacteria will build up on the tongue, gum, and cheeks. Remove that waste before eating or drinking to avoid swallowing it back into the gut. Try this morning routine to maximize all the other modalities discussed here. If you can't fit all this in, just pick a few and notice the benefits.

1. Open your mouth and inspect your tongue. If it has a gray or black coating, you have excess Vata. A yellow coating means too much Pitta. A whitish coating is excessive Kapha. The coating can help you discern what is out of balance. If you are taking medication, that may be the culprit, or it is eating food that has a negative impact on your health.

2. Use a metal or copper tongue scraper to clean this coating off your tongue. Grasp the ends and place it as far back on your tongue as possible, press firmly, and scrape forward. Do this three or four times, and rinse the scraper. If there is a heavy, thick coating on the scraper, do it a few more times.

3. Brush your teeth with an Ayurvedic herbal toothpaste, one containing only natural cleansers, or neem-based toothpaste or powders. Popular conventional brands contain chemicals, preservatives, and sweeteners. Brush the natural way. A pea-sized amount of toothpaste on your brush is all you need.

4. Take a tablespoon (15 ml) of sesame seed or coconut oil and hold it in your mouth for 10 to 15 minutes. Swish gently and pull between your teeth and gums. This is called oil pulling. When done, spit the oil into a trash can, not your sink (it will clog). Notice it is viscous as it has pulled bacteria out of your cheeks, tongue, and gums.

5. Take another tablespoon (15 ml) of oil and gargle with it, three or four times, and spit into the trash. Rinse with a pinch of baking soda in 2 ounces (59 ml) of water if you want to get the oil taste out of your mouth, but it's not necessary.

6. Now you are set for the day. The thin coating of oil that remains in the mouth is antimicrobial and will protect your teeth and gums from bad bacteria.

7. In the evening, floss your teeth with a neem-infused, mint-coated, or regular dental floss. Brush with your preferred toothpaste. A good trick is to brush after dinner so that you won't eat anymore!

Condition: Bad Breath

Poor food choices and weak agni (digestive fire) lead to bad breath. When food is not digested properly, it becomes a toxic residue called *ama*. This ama may be in your gut, liver, colon, intestines, and even your cheeks, gums, and tongue, resulting in breath that smells putrid. If your digestive fires are low, food will ferment and rot in your gut. The cure for bad breath is to stoke your digestive fires, digest your food completely after each meal, and clean the mouth properly.

FOOD

- Balance your pH. We often wake up acidic, so we want to bring the system back to basic, which is a balance between acid and alkaline. Too much acid can cause damage to the kidneys and other organs and an imbalance in the blood. If we had not-so-healthy food the day before, we may wake up too acidic. It's important to keep the pH balanced to function at the optimal levels. Begin your day with a cup of warm water with a squeeze of lemon or lime, or ½ teaspoon of apple cider vinegar. This will act to balance the pH in your system.

- Avoid dairy. This includes yogurt, milk, cheese, and butter. Ghee is not a problem as the milk solids have been removed.

- Eat only cooked foods. Cooking your food makes it easier to digest. Bake, poach, sauté, and roast. Don't fry or grill over high heat; both create a chemical called acrylamide, which is cancerous. Avoid microwaving, as it kills nutrients in the food.

- Eat a simple diet. Center your diet around healthy ingredients. Make sure to get enough fiber and carbs through beans, grains, and greens.

- Never have iced drinks or cold food, as these will extinguish the digestive fires. Reheat food on the stove or in the oven, or allow cold foods to come to room temperature before consuming.

- Ignite your agni. Eat a slice of fresh ginger with a bit of lime or lemon juice and a few grains of salt before a meal.

- Only sip water or a warm drink with your meal. If you drink too much water or liquids with meals, you wash away your saliva. Saliva is a natural barrier to harmful microbes and bacteria.

- Don't eat late. Always have your last meal at least 3 hours before you go to bed.

LIFESTYLE

- Breathe through your nose. Mouth breathing is a cause of bad breath. Air inhaled through the nose passes through a filtration process, and inhaling through the mouth does not provide that cleanse. Breathing through the mouth kills the good bacteria, resulting in not only bad breath, but in gingivitis, tooth decay, and even bone deformities. Look for mouth tape to close the mouth at night to train yourself to breathe through your nose exclusively. Only use tape designed for this practice.

- Practice sheetali breathing. See page 174 for details. This practice will cool and freshen the breath.

- Follow the practices for good oral care detailed on page 92.

APOTHECARY

- Chew a small handful of roasted fennel seeds or one or two cardamom seeds after meals. This will aid digestion and freshen breath.

- Place one or two drops of clove oil or tea tree oil on your finger and massage your gums once a day. Spit out any excess. Both are antibacterial and antifungal.

- Rinse your mouth with a simple solution of baking soda and water. Use ½ teaspoon in 2 to 3 ounces (60 to 90 ml) of warm water.

- Neem is antifungal, antimicrobial, and antibacterial and can help to rebuild healthy tissues. Use neem toothpaste and neem sticks. Chew on the stick until you split the bark, then rub the stick all over your teeth and gums.

- Drink 2 tablespoons (30 ml) of aloe vera juice every morning. Aloe cleanses the gut, which may be the source of your bad breath.

- Coconut oil is antimicrobial and will help you have fresh breath. Oil pull with coconut oil daily. Place 1 tablespoon (15 g) of coconut oil in your mouth, allow it to melt, and slowly swish and pull it through your gums and teeth for 15 to 20 minutes. Spit the oil into the trash when you are done.

Condition: High Cholesterol

For some people, high cholesterol is inherited. For others, it is caused by their food choices. Stress also raises cholesterol. The ancient Ayurvedic texts don't use the word "cholesterol"; rather, they look at fat or adipose tissue (called *meda dhatu* in Sanskrit). Meda dhatu is one of the seven dhatus, which means "tissues" in Sanskrit (see page 14), that make up our constitution. In modern Ayurveda, fat tissue gives us an indication of what is happening in the body, along with the LDL and HDL numbers. But it's the triglycerides that we really rely on.

Before I began practicing Ayurveda, my cholesterol was 240. The ratio between the HDL (the good one) and LDL (the bad one) was decent, but the overall count was too high. In Ayurveda, we use numbers and measurements as guidelines; I was about fifty pounds overweight, and the weight, on top of the high cholesterol, was troublesome. In conjunction with my weight loss, my cholesterol plummeted to 160. The result was astonishing—eighty points lower on my cholesterol. If I wasn't already a believer, I became one then!

Your Triglyceride/HDL Ratio

Extra, unused calories in the body are converted to triglycerides. If you overeat and your body has no use for the extra food, your triglyceride number will be high. And it's no coincidence that as you lose weight (if you have weight to lose), your triglyceride number decreases.

According to Dr. John Douillard, a longtime Ayurvedic practitioner, author, and speaker, the triglyceride/HDL ratio is where we need to focus our attention. Look at a recent blood cholesterol test, and divide the triglycerides by the HDL number to get your triglyceride/HDL ratio. Studies have shown that the lower your number the less likely you are to have cardiovascular issues. A number higher than 3 indicates a problem, and 2 is a good number, indicating a low risk. If you are looking strictly at your LDL and HDL, try to keep your LDL lower than 100 mg and your HDL above 60 mg. HDL is the good one: H = Happy. And in LDL, the L stands for Lousy.

Remember cholesterol is essential to our bodies and performs many important functions. If you are overweight, your cholesterol ratio may or may not be high, but it is important to pay attention and notice any changes. If you are underweight, you may or may not have enough cholesterol. Again, watch your numbers and aim for a healthy ratio by following the guidelines.

FOOD

- Reduce sugar. Basically, sugar turns to fat and fat raises your triglycerides and causes other damage. When there is too much simple sugar in the blood, it will glycate, meaning the sugar will attach to amino acids and proteins and become a sticky compound. Having something sticky in your bloodstream is not a good sign. Say no to sugar—white, brown, and even raw—it's all the same. Read labels and pay attention to how much processed sugar is in your food.

- Use natural sweeteners like raw honey, jaggery, or Sucanat (which stands for sugar cane natural). These are good alternatives to processed sugar. You may also try dates, molasses, maple syrup, pumpkin puree, yacon, agave nectar, stevia, coconut palm sugar, Florida crystals, and fruit jams and pulps as alternatives.

- Eat fatty fish, which is high in omega-3 fatty acids. Wild-caught mackerel, herring, tuna, salmon, sardines, anchovies, and trout are good sources of omegas.

Wild-Caught Fish

Eat 8 ounces (225 g) of fish two to three times a week. Bake, poach, or sauté, but don't fry. Canned fish that is wild caught and less expensive can be just as good; carefully read the labels to make sure the wild catches are sustainable. Farmed fish does not contain the same amount of nutrients, is less beneficial overall, and is cruel to the fish. Caution: Pregnant and nursing women should be aware of possible mercury content in wild-caught fish and not eat too much. Speak to your doctor or practitioner.

- Eat cholesterol-reducing foods. Most of the following foods are high in soluble fiber, which slows absorption of sugar and helps to wash away impurities and toxins. Plus, they are full of minerals, nutrients, vitamins, and many cholesterol-busting properties. Enjoy more oatmeal, whole grains (e.g., barley, quinoa, amaranth, and brown rice), beans, lentils, nuts, and seeds, fruits (e.g., apples, pears, bananas, kiwi, and berries), tofu, edamame, avocados, vegetables (e.g., eggplant and okra), grass-fed whey protein, olive oil, ghee, and green tea.

- Be moderate with alcohol. In the end, alcohol turns to sugar. Drinking also lowers inhibitions, causing you to eat more than you need to, usually late at night!

- Avoid foods high in saturated fats (solid fats) such as lard, butter, cream, hard cheese, beef, and pork. Read labels and avoid products with trans fats, hydrated or partially hydrogenated vegetable oil, hydrolyzed vegetable oil, and partially hydrolyzed vegetable oil. These are man-made and cannot be digested by the body. They actually cause damage and many companies are removing them from their products.

LIFESTYLE

- Reduce stress. Stress does horrible things to the body, and elevating bad cholesterol is one of them. A good way to learn how to reduce stress is to let go of the past and live more in the present moment, which may be easier said than done. Holding on to regrets, guilt, and shame do extreme harm to the mind and body. Meditation, exercise, or even petting and gazing into the eyes of a dog, horse, or animal you love helps immensely. Bird-watching or looking at fish in a pond or aquarium is also calming. Find a stress reduction path that works for you and incorporate it into your daily routine.

- Eat meals on a regular schedule. The body and mind function best when they know they are going to be fed. Two to three meals a day suits most people; avoid snacking, and eat only when hungry.

- Incorporate exercise and movement into your routine. Ideally, exercise every day; even bits throughout the day for a total of 30 minutes to one hour will make a difference. A combination of aerobics (e.g., swimming, walking, or jogging), using weights, and stretching, like yoga, will produce the best results.

- Quit smoking. And avoid being around people who are smoking—including vaping.

- Sleep at regular hours. If your work permits it, sleep on a regular schedule: 10 p.m. to bed and rise at 6 or 7 a.m. Don't sleep during the day as that disrupts the natural circadian cycle.

APOTHECARY

- *Amalaki* is an Indian fruit that has the highest amount of vitamin C compared to other fruits and vegetables and has been shown to keep blood sugar and cholesterol at healthy levels. Studies show it actually lowers triglycerides and LDL and raises HDL. The fruit is found at Indian stores or taken as a supplement. Eat one or two fruits a day if you can get them (preferred), or take the tablets, one or two a day with food. There are no contraindications.

- *Shilajit*, take two tablets once a day. Shalajit is a mineral resin that cleanses the blood and strengthens many organs in the body and reduces LDL while supporting HDL. Avoid if you have hypoglycemia or are pregnant.

- Guggulu, take ¼ teaspoon of the powder in 4 to 6 ounces (118 to 177 ml) of warm water once a day. Guggulu, a resin from tree bark most commonly found in India, is said to scrape toxins out of the body, including LDL, to balance your cholesterol. As a scraper, it's also excellent for weight loss and removing excess Kapha. Do not take if nursing or pregnant.

- Psyllium husk (insoluble fiber), take 1 or 2 teaspoons (5 to 10 g) once a day, with 8 ounces (235 ml) of water. Mix well and drink immediately.

Vata

Pitta

Kapha

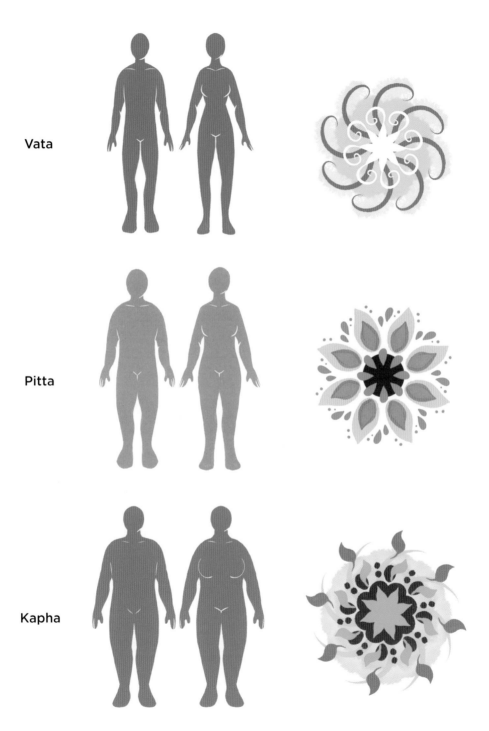

Doshas and Healthy Weight

Each dosha has a weight where they are healthiest. Vata-types really suffer if overweight, as they don't have the bone structure to bear it. Pitta-types function best at a medium weight, not too skinny and not too heavy. Kapha-types suffer if they are too thin and have difficulty maintaining a low weight naturally. Kapha weight is on the higher end of normal.

Notice where your body is most comfortable and where your guideline numbers, such as cholesterol, fall into place. LDL levels in the blood decrease as you lose weight. We do not rely on body mass index (BMI) numbers in Ayurveda, as they do not take individual constitutions into account; BMI gives you an idea, but it might create stress and anxiety. Talk to an Ayurvedic practitioner about the right doshic weight for you.

Condition: Dehydration

Beyond feeling thirsty, dehydration can affect your body in many different ways. It may make you confused and disoriented. Your body may be hot to the touch, and your lips and skin may become dry and cracked in severe cases. You may stop sweating, urine can become dark yellow, or you could become unable to urinate altogether. You might feel very tired, and in extreme cases, dehydration can cause you to faint and even die.

If you are dehydrated, the nutrients in your food cannot be absorbed and digested properly and will not nourish your gut, tissues, blood, bones, or cells. Dehydration is also one of the main causes of constipation. Feces and urine are two ways our body rids itself of toxins, and if not properly hydrated, the body can't detox and will poison itself.

Climate Change and Dehydration

With climate change, the earth is experiencing areas of extreme heat for longer durations than ever seen before. Many places do not have enough drinking water. In some towns and cities, the nighttime temperature is not much cooler than the daytime temperature, offering little relief. This creates what's called the wet lightbulb effect, when the heat and humidity exceed the temperature of the body, so that sweating provides no relief. This extremely dangerous condition can be fatal.

The climate crisis is creating enormous damage to the earth and its inhabitants. We need to remain vigilant as we seek ways to survive. Now, more than ever, we must be aware of our surroundings and be prepared for the extremes, including dehydration. At some point, consuming water and cooling down are not enough or may not even be an option, and you may need medical intervention.

Ayurveda says that if you are of normal weight, you should drink half your weight, in ounces of water, every day. So, if you weigh 150 pounds (68 kg), drink 75 ounces (2.2 L) of water a day. You may need more or less depending on your activity level and where you are in the world. If you are overweight, drink a bit less. Excess weight is Kapha, which is earth and water, so we avoid adding more water than necessary to Kapha.

FOOD

- Many foods and seeds have hydrating qualities. Chia and flaxseeds, when soaked, create a gel that your body will readily absorb. Soak 1 tablespoon (15 g) of seeds for about 20 minutes. They will become gelatinous. Add this to yogurt or over cereal, stir it into soup, or add it to a smoothie.

Hydrating Foods

Zucchini, squash, green beans, lettuce, celery, watercress, mushrooms, and okra all have high water content. Cruciferous vegetables, such as broccoli and cauliflower, fall into this category as well. Add in some sweet juicy plums, peaches, kiwis, mangoes, and nectarines too. These foods deliver the right amount of minerals and water to your cells and tissues, resulting in a well-hydrated body.

- Watery veggies are a must on hot days and during dry seasons, such as fall and early winter. Look for fruits and vegetables that have the highest water content and choose the freshest (plump, not shriveled) or go for frozen. If they have been sitting on a store shelf or trucked across the country (or the world), the produce may have dehydrated.

- Eat a good assortment of prebiotic and probiotic foods to feed your gut microbiome (see page 89). Do not drink caffeinated drinks or alcohol when you are dehydrated.

LIFESTYLE

- Avoid exercising in the heat of the day when your body may sweat out more fluid than it can replenish. Overexercising in a heated gym or doing hot yoga is excessive. Moderation is the best.

- Wear light-colored, loose, organic cotton or linen so that your skin can breathe.

- Sip water throughout the day to stay hydrated consistently. Carry a container with you at all times in all climates. Even in winter, heated homes, offices, and shopping malls are dehydrating.

Extreme Hydration Smoothie

Hydrate and replenish with this tasty, nutritious drink.

- ½ cup (120 ml) coconut milk
- 2 teaspoons (14 g) rose petal jam
- ⅓ cup (13 g) fresh basil leaves
- ¾ cup (113 g) fresh or frozen blackberries
- Juice from ½ a lime
- ½ teaspoon flaxseed oil
- Pinch of sea salt
- Splash of apple cider vinegar
- 1 cup (235 ml) filtered water

Combine all the ingredients in a high-powered blender. Enjoy immediately, or store in an airtight jar in the fridge for up to 1 day.

APOTHECARY

- Try this Ayurvedic remedy for keeping you hydrated or when you feel excessively thirsty: Take 16 ounces (455 ml) of water and add 1 teaspoon of Sucanat or jaggery (or any of the natural sugars), a pinch of sea salt, and a squeeze of lime juice. Sip this throughout the day.

- Massage your skin with coconut oil to cool down the body from the outside and sip unsweetened coconut water to replenish the inside.

- Soak ¼ teaspoon each of coriander, chia seeds, and flaxseeds in 12 ounces (340 ml) of warm water for 15 minutes. Strain and drink.

Condition: Gastroesophageal Reflux Disease (GERD) / Acid Reflux and Heartburn

It is reported that more than 40 percent of the US population has some form of heartburn. GERD, reflux, and heartburn share similar symptoms, including a burning sensation in your esophagus and chest, difficulty swallowing, coughing when you eat, and, in some cases, vomiting due to reflux of the stomach acids. The symptoms worsen when lying down or bending over.

Reflux happens on a full or empty stomach. This is because the valve between the stomach and esophagus is not closing properly. Too much food pushes acid out; too little food and the overproduction of acid will cause it to come back up into the esophagus.

This burning feeling is connected to Pitta Dosha. GERD is too much fire, or acid, in the belly. The fire is necessary to digest food properly, but it is out of control if you have heartburn symptoms. Foods that are processed, hot, spicy, fried, or made with unhealthy oils all create excess fire. It may be tricky to find the right balance.

GERD, reflux, and heartburn may also be caused by too much heat in the mind—stress, anxiety, anger, frustration, and impatience. Remember that the brain and the gut are connected via the vagus nerve. These remedies are not only to heal GERD, but to prevent it in the first place.

FOOD

- Eat two to three meals a day, with no snacks in between, so your gut knows when to expect food and when to make hydrochloric acid. If you snack throughout the day, you are producing copious amounts of acid all day long. A meal is about two handfuls of food. Do not overeat. When you burp, you are full. Put the fork or spoon down and push the plate away.

- Reduce consumption of hot, spicy food and drink, red wine, and alcoholic drinks. Choose white wine or beer instead. Riesling or any sweet wine can be smoother, but don't overdo it. Stick to one serving of alcohol a day, maybe two to three days a week. If you are going through a bad period of reflux or GERD, cut it out completely.

- Don't use ice. The cold tamps out the natural digestive fires and puts the stomach in overdrive to create more juices to break down the food.

- Avoid sour and acidic foods, such as tomatoes, eggplant, peppers, lemon, soda, aged cheese, red meat, and grilled and processed foods.

- Eat a light dinner, at least 3 hours before bed. Easy-to-digest, light foods include soups, cooked vegetables, and grains, like rice or quinoa. Eat your meals in a comfortable setting, away from TV, radio, or stressful conversations.

- Reduce or eliminate coffee. Drink decaf or herbal tea instead.

Balancing Teas

Some anti-inflammatory and acid-reducing/alkaline herbal teas may help remedy GERD, reflux, or heartburn. Try one of the following:

- Chicory: soothing to the gut
- Peppermint: works to enhance digestion for some (but not everyone); brew it light
- Ginger: works well for most people to regulate digestive acids
- Licorice: soothes the lining of the stomach; avoid if pregnant
- Roasted fennel seeds: steep in boiling water for cooling effects and to help with excess acid
- Chamomile: calms the tissues of the stomach and soothes the mind
- Marshmallow: coats the stomach and reduces overproduction of acids

LIFESTYLE

- Promote digestion by sleeping on your left side. This position supports your organs and reduces the risk of acid escaping into the esophagus.

- Raise your head with an extra pillow, or if you have a bed with an adjustable frame, raise the head to a comfortable level.

- Breathe deeply and evenly as you move toward sleep, using the cooling breath sheetali (see page 174), sipping cool air through a rolled tongue and exhaling through your nose. If you cannot roll your tongue, just purse your lips and inhale, then exhale through the nose.

- Get to sleep by 10 p.m., which is the time of night the metabolic juices begin to break down all you took in during the day.

Digestive Visualization

Visualize the digestive process taking place, the valve closing properly between the stomach and the esophagus. See the fire in the belly cooling down. Allow your thoughts to gravitate toward cool scenes and cleansing, healing waters. Notice what emotions arise when you feel reflux or heartburn. Is it anger or frustration? Resentment? Impatience? Try to find the emotion(s) and meditate on that, without allowing them to take over your mind. By noting without attachment, begin to diffuse the feelings. Place your awareness on your gut—this is where our happy hormones come from. Imagine your gut bathed in feel-good hormones to balance and harmonize your digestive fires, reaching up into your brain. Feel the negative emotions wash away, leaving behind a healthy gut to receive, metabolize, and transform food and emotions that will fully nourish you.

- Quit smoking and vaping. Immediately. And quit soda and sparkling water too. Immediately.

- Move. If you find yourself winded after just 5 or 10 minutes of movement, pull back and breathe normally through your nose. Slowly build up until you are breathing comfortably in and out through your nose when exercising.

- Reduce stress and find healthy ways to cope with unwanted, negative, hurtful feelings and emotions with mindfulness practices and visualizations.

- Wear loose-fitting clothes. Avoid tight underwear and bras, jeans, and anything that makes you suck your tummy in to zip or button up. This doesn't mean that you should keep buying larger clothes. If you need to lose weight, read the section on page 111.

APOTHECARY

- Put a pinch of baking soda into about 4 ounces (115 ml) of water and drink all at once. This will alkalinize the acid in the stomach. This is a once-in-a-while cure, maybe once or twice a week.

- A traditional Ayurvedic spice mixture called *Avipattikar churna* is ideal for cooling the stomach. It contains fifteen herbs, including Indian jalap root, cardamom, clove, ginger, black pepper, cinnamon, and other Ayurvedic herbs. Combine ½ teaspoon of the mixture with warm water and drink once or twice a day. Take for as long as needed, but please address the root causes so that you do not need to take digestive aids forever.

- Chew on a small handful of roasted fennel seeds. This is why you always see a dish of these at the door when you leave an Indian restaurant. They cool the stomach and promote digestion.

- Rub the belly with coconut or castor oil when feeling discomfort. The massage and cooling oil will help to reduce feelings of reflux. Use a drop of sandalwood oil, or eucalyptus for even more cooling sensations. Rub your palm across the belly in a clockwise motion, the same direction as peristalsis, the flow of digestion through the gastrointestinal tract.

It's important to know that GERD, reflux, and other intestinal issues that cause acid to back up into your esophagus and mouth are serious. The acid causes damage and erosion and even bleeding. If you are experiencing serious symptoms, please see your doctor. Conventional medicine, such as a proton pump inhibitor, for a period of time, may be necessary while you heal and make the lifestyle changes outlined here.

Case Study in Reflux

I had a client, Claire, a forty-eight-year-old woman, who was suffering from intense reflux throughout the day, even on an empty stomach and especially when she went to bed. After a thorough intake, we uncovered many issues, including hot flashes, intense flares of anger at real and perceived injustices, dissatisfaction and disappointments, and an overall feeling that she missed the boat on her life. An aspiring actress in her twenties, she met a man, married, and had twins within a few years of landing in Hollywood. While she loved her family, she had harbored resentment and discontentment about the career she left—for nearly twenty-five years!

She had an aha moment when I pointed this out to her. Her stomach was gurgling with these stressors nearly all the time. No wonder she had frequent bouts of diarrhea followed by days of constipation, signs of nutrient malabsorption. Along with the food and drink guidelines in this chapter, I recommended that she find ways to express her creative side. Her longing to be on the stage was so great, but she could just never see a way to make it happen. We looked into local acting classes and dinner theaters, and before long, she joined a class and was auditioning for plays. Her home life transformed, and her family was so excited to watch her finally take the stage.

And, her reflux went away. She told me she sleeps on her left side, eats dinner at least 3 hours before bed, and avoids snacking, alcohol, and spicy food. I believe her longing to express herself helped her change her life, and just like that, resentment, anger, frustration, and blame went away—along with an overly acidic stomach.

Weight Loss

Attaining and maintaining your proper weight is a major factor in eliminating diseases and digestive issues, as well as improving sleep. To lose weight, follow a Kapha-reducing plan. That means:

- Eat two meals a day, the largest meal of the day between 10 a.m. and 2 p.m. Eat a light dinner.
- Do not eat anything at all after 7 p.m.
- Sip water and herbal tea throughout the day.
- Take one triphala tablet after every meal, or two before bed, for regular bowel movements and a colon cleanse.
- Move your body somehow, some way, every day. A brisk walk outside is the very best. Or a mix of stretching, aerobic, and strengthening exercise, at least 30 minutes every other day. Do a more intense workout one or two days a week, for at least 30 minutes.
- Avoid dairy, wheat, and sugar.
- Eat more greens, grains, and beans.
- Avoid ALL processed food. No fast food. No food with more than seven ingredients on the label.
- No soda or carbonated drinks (kombucha is okay).
- Reduce alcohol to one drink, once or twice a week. None at all works too. A good substitute for a drink is kombucha or KeVita, which is a water-based kefir drink. They are naturally sweet and fill your gut with good bacteria.
- Your largest meal is lunch.
- Your smallest meal is dinner.
- No food AT ALL after dinner.
- No snacks AT ALL. Eat your food at your meals.
- Each meal is two handfuls of food, which is a small bowl.
- If you are not hungry, don't eat.
- Go to sleep by 10 p.m. or 11 p.m. and wake up by or before 7 a.m.
- You can lose weight at a good steady pace. No matter your age or gender.

Condition: Irritable Bowel Syndrome (IBS)

IBS is the name given to a host of issues in the belly and bowels. The symptoms vary from person to person and even within the same person from week to week or day to day. They include constipation or diarrhea; stomach pains or cramps, sometimes worse after meals and alleviated after a bowel movement; gas or bloating; mucus in the stool; feeling of incomplete bowel movement; not being able to handle certain foods; exhaustion; anxiety; headaches; depression; indigestion. Typically, IBS can be a lifelong issue with flare-ups lasting a few weeks to six months before calming down again.

With such a wide variety of symptoms, doctors may sometimes just prescribe a laxative or an antidiarrheal. Some symptoms may be difficult to identify as IBS, and some physicians may prescribe an antidepressant to help ease the patient's stress and anxiety. Food is not always thoroughly addressed, and the patient may be left to wonder if it's all in their head.

Weak agni is the main culprit here. Food that is not properly digested leaves waste and toxins behind, which cause a doshic imbalance. Too much Vata, Pitta, or Kapha will increase many of the symptoms described above. The following remedies rid the body of toxins, support the gut microbiome, and balance the doshas.

FOOD

- All doshas should reduce fried and processed foods, red meat, dairy, oil (except for small amounts of ghee and olive oil), fatty foods, and hot spices (e.g., chiles, cayenne, hot curries).

- Consume high-fiber foods, including oatmeal; split mung beans or lentils (cooked with a pinch of hing); fruit, such as cooked apples or pears; berries and sweet, juicy fruits such as peaches, plums, watermelons; dates; and figs. If you notice adverse effects from these foods like gas and bloating, reduce or avoid them.

Hing

Hing, also known as *asafoetida*, is a spice derived from tree resin. It is often used in South Asian cooking to increase digestibility.

Bristol Stool Chart

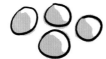

TYPE 1

Separate hard lumps
VERY CONSTIPATED

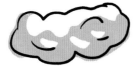

TYPE 2

Lumpy, sausage-like
SLIGHTLY CONSTIPATED

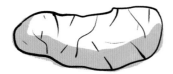

TYPE 3

Sausage shape, cracks in surface
NORMAL

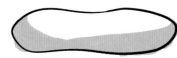

TYPE 4

Smooth, soft sausage or snake
NORMAL

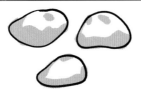

TYPE 5

Soft blobs, clear-cut edges
LACKING FIBER

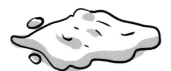

TYPE 6

Mushy, ragged edges
INFLAMMATION

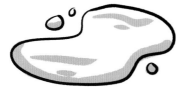

TYPE 7

Liquid, no solid pieces
INFLAMMATION AND DIARRHEA

Belly-Pacifying Kitchari

Kitchari is a *panacea* in Ayurvedic cuisine. The combination of ghee, spices, split yellow mung beans, and rice is not only a perfect meal, but it is soothing, easy to digest, and oh-so satisfying. Try adding seasonal vegetables to vary the ingredients and use all organic if possible. Eating kitchari for breakfast, lunch, and dinner for three to five days once a month is quite effective. Everything you need is in this bowl.

- ½ cup (113 g) split yellow mung beans/dahl
- ½ cup (93 g) white basmati rice
- 1–2 teaspoons (5 to 10 g) ghee
- 1 teaspoon black mustard seeds
- ½ teaspoon cumin seeds
- ½ teaspoon ground coriander
- ½ teaspoon ajwain seeds
- Pinch of hing (asafoetida)
- 1 teaspoon ground turmeric
- 1 small onion, chopped
- 1 small knob of fresh ginger, peeled and grated or minced
- 4–6 cups (940 ml to 1.4 L) water
- 1 or 2 seasonal vegetables, chopped (optional)
- Salt and freshly ground black pepper
- Greens
- 1 handful chopped fresh cilantro or parsley (optional)
- Ghee and Bragg's Liquid Aminos (optional)

Rinse the mung beans and rice together until the water runs relatively clear, should be two to three rinses. Fill the bowl with water and let them soak while you prepare the recipe, or up to 1 hour.

Make the *vagar* (oil/spice mix): (Have your exhaust fan on as the spices are strong). In an 8-quart (7.5 L) soup pot, heat the ghee over medium-high heat. Add the black mustard seeds. When they pop, add the cumin seeds, coriander, ajwain (aka Bishop's weed or carom seed), hing, and turmeric. Add the onions and ginger. Cook for 1 minute, or until aromatic. Spices burn quickly so make sure it does not begin to smoke. Lower the heat.

Drain the rice and mung beans and add them to the vagar. Mix until coated. Let that sit for a minute. Add the water and stir. Stir in the vegetables (if using). Cover, raise the heat and bring to a boil, then lower to a simmer.

Cook for 15 minutes, or until all the water is absorbed or the kitchari is the consistency you desire. More water makes it soupy, less water makes it more like a stew. Season with salt, pepper, and greens if desired. Stir well. Remove from the heat.

Place your portion in a large bowl (two handfuls) and top with cilantro or parsley (if using). Feel free to add a teaspoon of ghee as well as a dash of liquid aminos. To reheat, add a bit of water to the pot and cook over a medium heat until warm. Never microwave or freeze as that depletes the nutrients.

NOTE

Choose one or two seasonal vegetables, or none at all. Carrots and celery are always good. Try green beans or asparagus in spring, zucchini in summer, sweet potatoes or squash in fall or winter. It's always beneficial to toss a few handfuls of kale, spinach, or chard in at the end of cooking, just enough time to let them wilt, before serving.

Meditation for Belly Pain

Wear soft, neutral-colored, loose clothing and bras with no underwire. Find a quiet place where you won't be disturbed or distracted. Sit for 5 to 30 minutes a day, allowing your thoughts to roam without trying to control them. Just watch the thoughts and pain float by like clouds. Try not to hold on to any sensation, feeling, or emotion. Just notice it and let it pass.

Breathe normally. Let your belly be soft, no need to hold your stomach in as we have been conditioned to do. Your belly should expand on the inhale and contract on the exhale.

- Add foods on the probiotic and prebiotic list (page 89) to your diet. Introduce them slowly so that your gut builds up the enzymes to assimilate the new foods.

- Avoid hard, dry foods such as crackers, pretzels, and raw vegetables. Eat only easy-to-digest foods—your gut will tell you!

- Eat on a regular schedule, and do not overeat. The kitchen closes at 7 p.m., except for tea and water.

- Always hydrate. Drink plenty of room temperature water. Coconut or cucumber water in warm climates is great (unsweetened, of course). Sip herbal teas such as ginger or chamomile throughout the day. Avoid caffeine, carbonated drinks, and alcohol.

LIFESTYLE

- Relax. Activate the vagus nerve through deep, paced breathing: Inhale 4 seconds, hold 4 seconds, exhale 4 seconds—all through the nose.

- Move the body in ways to get rid of gas and bloating. Do seated twists, downward dog, cobra, and cat/cow poses.

- Eat a light dinner and get to bed by 10 p.m. so your body digests all the intake from the day and your system isn't overwhelmed.

APOTHECARY

- Drink aloe vera juice on an empty stomach—2 ounces (60 ml), twice a day. Buy the juice, not the gel you rub on your skin.

- Take one to two triphala (a blend of three Indian fruits) tablets before bed, with warm water. Try one tablet if you are having loose stools and two if you are constipated. You should notice a change in your bowel movements within a few days. Triphala detoxes, tones, and cleanses the colon, increasing the absorption of nutrients. There are no contraindications.

- Take Slippery Elm tablets—one or two in the morning, with food. This will help to calm a spastic stomach and relieve constipation. Slippery Elm bulks up stool and increases mucus to establish its passage is easy. Take the tablets at least 1 hour before medication as it coats the stomach and may decrease absorption of your medicine. There are no contraindications.

Condition: Gastric / Peptic Ulcer

Conventional Western medicine says that gastric (aka peptic) ulcers are caused by the *Helicobacter pylori* (which is commonly called *H. pylori*) bacteria or the overuse of NSAIDS such as ibuprofen, aspirin, and naproxen sodium. The bacteria and NSAIDS cause the stomach lining to weaken and tear, creating a painful sore. The mucosal layer, which is usually thick, will thin out if digestive acids erode the protective lining. As the acids eat away at the tissue, an ulcer appears in the intestines or the stomach.

In Ayurveda, we believe ulcers may be caused by bacteria and medicines, as well as Vata or Pitta being out of balance. As with most gut issues, the mind plays a starring role. Stress and anxiety, Ayurveda says, cause a thinning of the lining of the stomach. Excess acid is produced when we are stressed out, angry, impatient, or upset. This creates gastric imbalances and Pitta ulcers. Pitta ulcers lead to burning and gripping pain and cause reflux and low agni (digestive strength).

A Vata ulcer is caused by skipping meals, not eating on a proper schedule, eating tiny amounts, not having food in the stomach for long periods of time, and ignoring hunger. Because of the lack of food in the stomach, the acids build up and accumulate, increasing the likelihood of erosion of the stomach lining and tissues, causing an ulcer.

Gastric ulcers are difficult to diagnose as the symptoms are similar to those of heartburn and gastritis. Those symptoms include a burning sensation in the stomach, severe abdominal pain, nausea, vomiting, burping, blood in the stool, quick satiety, bloating, and weight loss. See your doctor or a gastroenterologist for the proper diagnosis. Along with conventional treatment, which may include antibiotics, use Ayurveda for support and to avoid a recurrence.

FOOD

- Avoid spicy and sour foods, including citrus, hot chiles, and peppers. Steer clear of fast food and fried foods, red meat, processed meats and snacks, and carbonated drinks. Stay away from red wine and coffee as they both irritate the stomach lining.

- Eat more blueberries, strawberries, raspberries, blackberries, apples, red grapes, bananas, green tea, kale, cabbage, carrots (and carrot juice), and leafy greens. Also include dark chocolate (at least 70 percent dark), 1 to 2 ounces (28 to 85 g), in your diet a day. These foods are high in polyphenols, which are healing for the gut.

- Raw honey is especially healing to the gut lining. Take 1 to 2 tablespoons (20 to 40 g) on an empty stomach, once a day. Manuka honey is highly effective. Remember to use only raw honey, as pasteurized honey is heated to a level that kills nutrients, minerals, and propolis.

- Review the prebiotic and probiotic food list (page 89) and incorporate them into your diet to help heal an ulcer.

- Try this garlic/milk mash to replenish the stomach lining. This ancient Ayurvedic recipe says to cook six medium-sized garlic cloves in 2 ounces (60 ml) of whole milk and 8 ounces (235 ml) of water. When the garlic is soft, mash it in the pot and keep cooking until the liquid is reduced to 2 ounces. Strain and drink the remaining liquid.

LIFESTYLE

- Quit smoking and don't be around others smoking or vaping. Smoke erodes the stomach lining.

- Meditate or practice breathing exercises, such as sheetali (page 174) and alternate nostril breathing (page 175). The idea is to calm down, reduce stress, and be happy or content.

- Eat three meals a day on a regular schedule. Dinner should be light but enough to fill your stomach. Remember that a meal is two handfuls of food. So, dinner could be a bowl of soup, rice and vegetables, or sautéed greens over grains and beans.

- Do not skip meals, even if you are overweight. Keep to the three meals, no snacks rule, which will help to balance out the production of gastric acids.

Replenishing Rice Kanji

A soothing, healing rice recipe, *kanji* is great for settling stomach acids and feeling nourished. Basically, this is rice that is cooked for a long time to break it down. It's a go-to dish for me whenever I am having gastric issues. It's easy to digest, nourishing, and surprisingly tasty. Kanji is thought to build a strong immune system, keep you healthy, and aid in recovery from many ailments.

- 1 cup (185 g) white rice (basmati and jasmine are good options)
- 5 cups (1.2 L) water
- Salt
- Pinch of ground turmeric, ground cumin, and ground ginger (optional)
- 1 teaspoon ghee (optional)

Rinse the rice two or three times under running water. Add it to a large pot with the water. Bring it to a boil over high heat, then lower the heat to a simmer with the cover slightly askew to let some steam out. Add salt to taste, and simmer for 30 minutes. Don't drain the water, that's very important!

After 30 minutes, it will be a thick rice soup. Stir in the spices and ghee (if using) or eat it plain. This is great for breakfast, lunch, and/or dinner.

NOTE

Do not use brown rice in this recipe. With the hull attached to the grain, brown rice is more difficult to digest than white rice. For this purpose, we suggest white to ease and aid digestion. There are many varieties of rice to choose from, so explore!

- Get enough sleep. For most people, this is 7 to 9 hours of good sleep, which has you feeling rested when you wake up. Your body needs to rest to repair.

- Wear nonrestrictive clothing. Loose waistbands are good. Women should avoid underwire bras. Don't wear any clothing that creates tension and restriction on the torso. All undergarments should allow freedom of motion for breath and intestinal movements.

APOTHECARY

- Cranberry capsules or gummies fight bacteria. Take one or two a day with or without food. You may also drink 1 cup (235 ml) of unsweetened cranberry juice instead.

- Mix ¼ teaspoon of licorice with a teaspoon of honey or a teaspoon of ghee. Drink two or three times a day. This will help to replenish the mucosal lining of the stomach. Avoid licorice if pregnant.

- Slippery Elm bark comes in tablets or powder and heals the stomach lining. Mix a teaspoon with hot water, or take two tablets once a day, with or without food.

- *Moringa* is known for treating gastrointestinal disorders and is antibacterial. Moringa seed pods may also be known as the Indian vegetable called drumstick, which can be found in Indian grocery stores. Moringa tea is widely available, as are moringa supplements. See the packaging for dosage. There are no contraindications.

- Turmeric will reduce inflammation and may fight *H. pylori*. Take as a supplement or use in your food—1 teaspoon a day. Make your own turmeric tea by adding ½ teaspoon of turmeric powder to 1½ cups (355 ml) of boiling water. Let it steep for 5 minutes before drinking.

- Roasted fennel seeds are great for balancing stomach acids. Chew on a small handful after each meal. Dry roast on a frying pan over medium heat for 3 minutes, or until aromatic.

- Ginger aids digestion and stokes the digestive juices. Eat a dime-sized piece of fresh ginger with a sprinkle of salt and a squeeze of lime juice about a half hour before a meal.

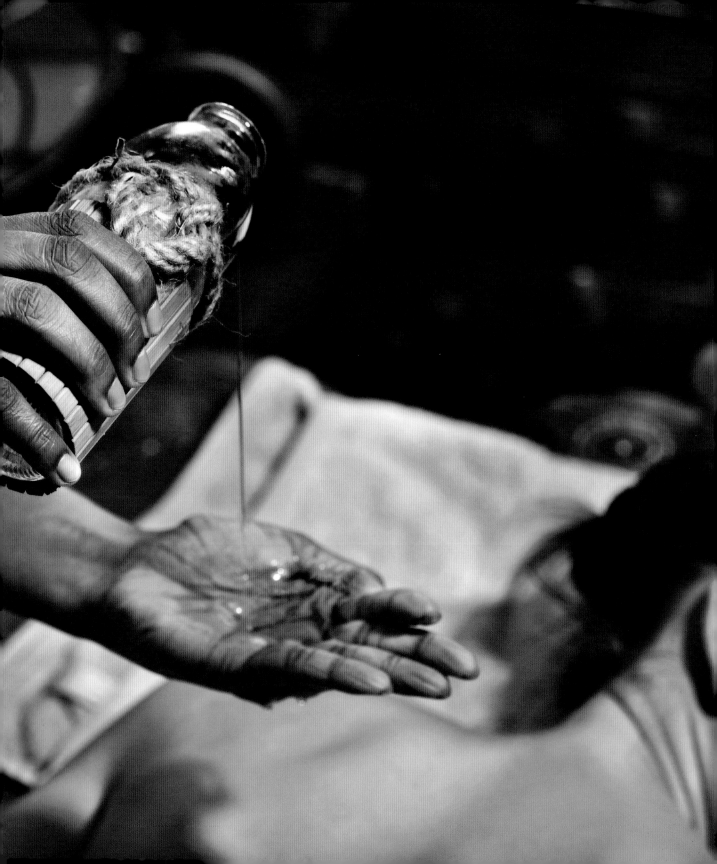

5

Skin:
The Body's Largest Organ

The general well-being of this all-encompassing organ relies
on the care of both the skin microbiome and the gut microbiome.
This means eat well and do less topically to disturb the good
bacterial layer, which is there for a reason: to nourish the skin and
create a foolproof barrier from toxins, incursions, invasions, and
other environmental assaults. Ayurveda is replete with oils, herbs,
and strategic ideas for replenishing lost moisture and elasticity, to
aids for supporting skin nutrition from the inside out.

You Really Are What You Eat

In Sanskrit we call the skin the *anamaya kosha*, meaning "the layer derived from food." What we consume and how we digest it shows up on the outside as either radiant skin, or sallow, patchy, dull, gray skin. When I began to practice Ayurveda, the word I heard most often from people was "glowing." "You are glowing," over and over again. It was a product of everything we have been talking about in these pages. The benefits pay off not only in great health, a robust immune system, and increased longevity, but you also look fantastic! Who wouldn't want that at any age? Ayurvedic practices protect and nourish our bodies inside and out.

Throughout our lives we may face many skin issues that arise at different times, including acne, rashes, hives, dryness, and oiliness. Many of these issues surface from hormonal changes. Other problems may come from accidents such as burns and cuts. Others are just from living a full life, like wrinkles and laugh lines. Food, salves, balms, and best practices for helping out your skin are all discussed here.

FOOD: THE GUT MAKES THE SKIN

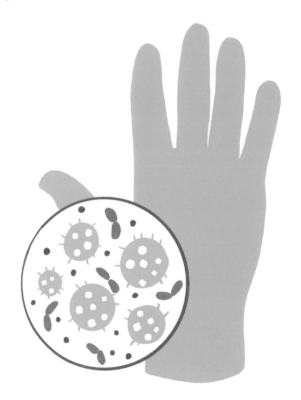

- Get your omega-3s. For beautiful skin, make sure your diet is rich in omega-3 fatty acids such as those found in fish (e.g., salmon and mackerel), nuts and seeds (e.g., walnuts and sunflower seeds), vegetables (e.g., beets and kale), fruits (e.g., avocados, strawberries, and blueberries), and even dark chocolate.

- Avoid junk food. What goes in your mouth is going to show up on the outside sooner or later. Let go of sugary, salty, or prepackaged foods. You simply cannot cheat on great-looking skin.

LIFESTYLE: DRESSING FOR PROTECTION AND BEAUTY

- Allow the skin to breathe. Wear clothes made of natural fibers that fit loose and comfortably. Sleep either naked or in loose PJs. Forgo underwear. Let the entire body breathe.

- Make sure your pillowcase is washed in natural plant-based detergent and is made from natural, organic fibers like hemp or cotton.

APOTHECARY: LESS IS MORE

- Avoid overwashing your skin. Leave the microbiome alone as much as possible. Removing the microbiome will cause your skin to overproduce oils as it feels it is being assaulted, and it will try to replenish its natural state of being.

- Skip sunbathing. Instead, practice sun gazing at dawn and dusk. Look toward the sun when it is on the horizon for 5 to 10 seconds. Look away and back again several times. In the morning, this process will flood the body with light to wake us up. In the evening, the setting sun will encourage the production of melatonin to help us sleep. Never stare directly at the sun once it is over the horizon.

Condition: Acne

Typically a Pitta condition of too much heat and oil in the body, acne expresses itself on the skin: usually on the face, neck, chest, and back. It may come on at puberty or later in life when stress is present. Certain medications cause breakouts as well as diet, cosmetics, and topical creams. The suggested practice will remove excess heat, support the system in detoxifying (primarily the liver, lymph, and blood), and promote hydration.

FOOD

- Eat a Pitta-reducing diet: Avoid hot, spicy, and fried foods, which will only exacerbate the problem.

- Eat foods that naturally hydrate with cooling juices, such as coconut, celery, cucumbers, romaine, and juicy fruits. Eat leafy greens every day to hydrate and detoxify.

- Avoid alcohol and spirits especially when you have an outbreak. Alcohol creates a lot of heat, which will erupt on your skin. A good substitute for a drink is kombucha or KeVita, which is a water-based kefir drink.

LIFESTYLE

- De-stress. Stress creates hormonal surges that erupt on the skin, causing red patches, itching or burning hives, acne, and even dry patches. By getting the hormones under control, the skin stays calm, cool, and collected. Do this by learning to meditate, or even just sitting still for 5 or 10 minutes a day. Meditation doesn't need to be a rigid practice. Focus on breathing. You may look at a candle, a flower, or a photo of a beautiful scene. Let go. Relax.

- If you have long hair, pull it off your face at all times. The oils and chemicals from shampoos, gels, and other products will aggravate the skin, face, and neck.

- After sweating or exercising, splash your face with water and pat dry. Don't wash your face with cleanser every time you sweat. Water will rinse away the toxins. Soap will exacerbate the problems.

APOTHECARY

- Never scrub, rub, or exfoliate as that will only add to the problem. Avoid harsh chemicals, treatments, and peels. This causes an overproduction of oil, creating clogging in the sebaceous glands, resulting in more acne.

- Several Ayurvedic companies have tablets containing herbs to support healing and maintain healthy skin. Look for the following:

  » *Manjistha* is the ultimate herb for a healthy complexion, balancing heat and supporting detoxification of the liver and kidneys. Mix ¼ teaspoon of powder into a small amount of warm water and drink once or twice a day, after food. There are no contraindications.

  » Neem repairs and maintains healthy skin. Take two tablets once a day after food. Avoid if pregnant or nursing or if you have hypoglycemia.

  » Turmeric supports skin and nourishes the tissues, creating that healthy glow. Take a turmeric tablet once or twice a day or add at least 1 teaspoon a day to food, ideally tempered in oil. Avoid the tablets if you are pregnant or have gallstones.

Condition: Sunburn

When I was kid growing up in the seventies, a summer ritual with my sisters was to take a two-sided record album cover, wrap it with tinfoil, cover ourselves with baby oil, and sit in the backyard with the foil reflecting the sun on our faces. We would do this for hours and we had a sunlamp for the winter months. Sometimes I wonder how I got out of childhood alive, and with decent skin! I can't even imagine the damage that my sisters and I did to our skin, but we somehow survived with no major disasters. Maybe it was genetic.

Of course, now we all know better and wouldn't even think of putting our faces in the sun without a natural sunscreen and certainly not in the middle of the day. A serious sunburn causes blistering, fever, vomiting, dehydration, and shaking. If you are displaying any of these symptoms, call your doctor. But many people still risk it, aching for that tanned "healthy" look. They use tanning beds and spray-on tans too. Let's get real. A tan does not in any way mean you are healthy. A tanning bed is known to cause cancer with both dangerous UVB and UVA rays, while tanning sprays and creams may contain harmful chemicals.

But we need the sun to live, to activate our circadian rhythm, and to produce vitamin D.

FOOD

- If you have sunburn, avoid all hot, spicy food, caffeine, and alcohol until you have recovered.

- Eat cooling foods such as cucumbers, coconut, fresh greens, cilantro, and sweet juicy fruits.

- Stay hydrated by sipping cool coconut water or regular water throughout the day.

LIFESTYLE

- Avoid being in direct sun from 10 a.m. to 3 p.m. Wear lightweight, light-colored clothes with long sleeves and long pants if you need to be out midday. Wear a wide-brimmed hat to protect your face, ears, and neck from damaging sun rays.

- Allow the sun to be on your face and limbs in the morning and late afternoon hours. This will help flood your body with natural vitamin D. Vitamin D is essential for strong bones, and to promote everything from a robust cardiovascular system to balancing sugars, elevating mood, and preventing cancer.

APOTHECARY

- When you are out in the sun, use a natural sunblock such as neem oil or coconut oil. Use neem that is in a carrier oil such as coconut, sesame, or sunflower. Make your own by adding five to ten drops of neem oil to 4 ounces (120 ml) of the carrier oil. Shake well. This will prevent bug bites as well.

- Use aloe vera gel on sunburned skin. Ancient Ayurveda also suggests using cream or goat or cow milk on sunburned skin. Soak a cloth or gauze in milk and lay it directly onto the skin.

- Mix equal parts sandalwood and turmeric powder with cool water and create a paste to apply directly to the skin. Be aware that this will stain your skin, clothes, and towels. Pure sandalwood powder is difficult to find. If you cannot locate it, just use turmeric.

- If you are craving a natural, healthy glow, attain it by eating well or you can buy it. You can find bronzing products that are plant-based and fair-trade.

Condition: Hives and Rashes

Hives, also known as urticaria, are a vexing symptom. They are easy to diagnose, but it's challenging to uncover the cause and find a cure. In Ayurveda we say that hives are cold taking over hot, so we must find the cause of each and create balance. Hives are called *sheetapitta* in Sanskrit—sheeta means cold, and pitta means hot.

Often, they appear and disappear on their own, sometimes showing up as white, pink, or red welts or bumps on the skin. They often burn, itch, or cause extreme discomfort. In Ayurveda our goal is to get to the root cause. After stripping away layer after layer of possible causes, such as allergens, detergents, medications, or food, we investigate psychological issues, stress, tension, and lifestyle choices. Usually, I peel back one thing at a time to help find the culprit—often it's a combination of factors, like food, drink, and lifestyle.

Sometimes the root cannot be identified and the hives are thought of as coming from an indeterminate cause. In rare cases hives result from thyroid problems or even cancer. If you have hives for longer than six weeks, make an appointment with your GP for blood and lab work.

FOOD

- Hives are hot, so remove all that is spicy, pungent, and acidic. This includes red wine, hot mustard, and red meat. Sour foods may cause hives as well. Avoid citrus, vinegar, and tart fruits like cherries and cranberries. Avoid acidic foods such as tomatoes, salsas, yogurt, and kimchi.

- Peanuts, eggs, nuts, and shellfish should be removed from the diet and brought back in slowly once the hives have disappeared to see if they may be the cause. Avoid all processed foods. The preservatives, dyes, and chemical flavorings wreak havoc on the body, causing hives and allergic reactions.

- Eat only warm and cooked food. Cold, raw foods will be difficult to digest and disrupt the system. Stick with plant-based milks while healing. Eat complex carbs, organic grains, split mung beans, and lentils. Sauté spices such as turmeric, fennel seed, and cumin in ghee and add them to your greens, beans, or grains.

- Drink plenty of warm water and stinging nettle tea, which will help to combat the allergens. Eat bitter foods, which are highly detoxifying, such as dandelion greens, cruciferous vegetables, raw cocoa powder, and green tea. Bitter gourd can be found in Indian and Asian food stores and is worth a try.

- Cut back on salt intake. Use cooling spices such as cardamom, cinnamon, fennel seed, and turmeric instead. Use raw honey instead of sugar. Excessive sugar intake is widely thought to cause hives. This includes cakes, cookies, and pastries.

- Stop smoking immediately, as the poisonous heated chemicals in the tobacco may erupt as skin rashes.

Eladi Tailam

Eladi Tailam is an oil blend of many Ayurvedic herbs. Studies show it to be highly effective for many skin disorders, including hives, acne, dark under-eye circles, and rashes. It is widely available from Ayurvedic companies. For hives, rashes, and itchy skin, use the Eladi Tailam that is prepared in sesame seed oil, as opposed to coconut oil. There are no contraindications and it is safe for children, but test on a small patch of skin first. Wait a few hours and make sure there is no allergic reaction. Apply once or twice a day.

LIFESTYLE

- Begin a meditation practice to calm the mind. Hives are mentally and physically aggravating. Even 5 minutes of sitting still once or twice a day helps the body heal. Sit quietly and focus on your breath. Use a mantra, calming words of your choice, on the in breath and out breath (through the nose) to keep you focused.

- It is advised not to sleep during the day. Ayurveda says this increases Kapha, which may play a role in the imbalance. If you must nap, do it sitting up rather than lying down, and for less than 20 minutes.

- Wear loose clothing made from natural fibers. If you have hives around your torso, waist, or genitals, you may want to avoid underwear, bras, and camisoles for a time.

- Bathe a few times a week in warm water, pat dry, and apply recommended oils. Do not use soaps or scrubs.

- Don't eat after 7 p.m. and go to sleep by 10 p.m. Wear a loose nightgown or shirt, or sleep naked on organic cotton or flannel sheets washed in plant-based detergent.

APOTHECARY

- Try coconut, neem, or mustard oil for a few days to see which brings you the most relief. Apply liberally all over the hives to help quell the outbreak.

- Triphala is known as a colon cleanser and toner, and a remover of toxins from the blood and tissues. Take two tablets before bed. If this causes loose bowels, take one tablet. If it causes constipation, make sure you drink a large glass of warm water when you take a tablet.

- Take neem tablets twice a day or mix ¼ teaspoon of neem powder in a small amount of warm water and drink twice a day, for four weeks, with or without food. Keep taking the tablets for an additional week or two, even if the rash clears up, to continue strengthening and cleaning the cells, blood, and tissues. Avoid neem if you are nursing or pregnant.

- Ashwagandha nourishes the entire mind/body, making it a wonderful supplement for the sometimes hard-to-diagnose hives issues. For hives, take two, with or without food, every day for at least four weeks. Ashwagandha has the added benefit of deeply relaxing the nervous system. Do not take if you are pregnant.

Condition: Dry Skin

When things get out of balance in the body, Vata is usually to blame. With dry skin, it's clearly a Vata disorder, but there are hints of Pitta too, especially if there is red, flaky, inflamed skin. The sebaceous glands in the face produce sebum, the layer of oil that protects the facial skin from damaging toxins. It keeps the skin moist, and in most environments, it is able to adjust the amount of oil produced to keep the skin healthy and glowing. Even in cold and dry or hot and dry climates, when working well, our skin should be well oiled with a healthy sheen.

For some reason, though, we scrub, rub, tug, and exfoliate, spending hundreds, if not thousands, of dollars on serums, soaps, and solutions that strip the skin of its natural oils and good bacterial microbiome. I'm here to tell you stop that! We wash too much and disturb the skin's ability to breathe, hydrate, and oil itself.

Dry skin is caused by aging, cold weather, harsh chemicals, a poor diet, and even bathing in hot water. You may notice dried cracked lips, wrinkles, itchiness, flakes of skin on your face, and perhaps even cracks that bleed. Legs and arms may have dry patches, especially on the elbows and knees. It may come and go, or be worse in cold and dry weather. Stress and not eating well can also make it worse.

Identifying the cause helps to repair the damage. Home remedies are often cheaper and more effective than anything on the market. And what you eat is just as important as what you use on your skin. Remember that the skin, in Sanskrit, is called the *anamaya kosha*, the layer derived from food. If the body is well fed, it is reflected on the skin.

FOOD

- Keep hydrated by drinking room temperature or warm water throughout the day. Drink consistently rather than having large amounts of liquids every few hours. Warmer water is more easily absorbed in the tissues than cold, iced drinks. Certain teas, such as chamomile, ginger, fenugreek, and lemongrass, are especially beneficial for the skin and complexion.

- Consume hydrating foods such as melon, cucumber, and coconut. Add chia and flaxseeds to your meals.

Eat Warm Food

To help remedy dry skin from the inside out, try eating a fruit compote with apples or pears. To make, boil a small pot of water, then add one chopped up apple or pear with a pinch of cinnamon or nutmeg. Bring to a boil, reduce to a simmer, and cook until the fruit is soft. Stir in a spoonful of raw honey or maple syrup if you want it sweeter. Eat the fruit and drink the liquid.

- Eat soup in cold months, at least once a day. All food should be warm. It is especially important in winter that food be cooked and warm so that the body does not need to generate more heat to digest. Cold food needs to be warmed up in the gut to break it down and digest. In the winter, we need to conserve that energy to keep the rest of the body warm.

- Use ghee, coconut, sesame, and avocado oil for roasting vegetables, sautéing greens, or adding to rice and grains. Olive oil becomes rancid when exposed to high heat; add it to cooked foods, such as pasta or vegetables, or use it on a low or medium heat.

- Enjoy unctuous foods such as avocado, sweet potatoes, yams, and bananas. Butter, whole milk, and ghee are good choices. Nuts are great and full of fat and nutrients. Try soaking the nuts for an hour or overnight, to make them even more digestible.

- Avoid Vata-provoking foods that are frozen, cold, or dry, such as crackers, pretzels, cold cereals, uncooked vegetables, as well as Brussels sprouts, mushrooms, raw onions, and tomatoes.

LIFESTYLE

- Sleep is a pillar of Ayurveda: When we sleep, the body repairs itself, including the skin. Get to sleep by 10 p.m., and sleep for 7 to 9 hours.

- Reduce showers and baths until they are necessary. Oil the body before or after. Use warm to lukewarm water. Hot water exacerbates dry skin conditions. Use a mild soap just in the areas you need to, like under the arms and breasts, the groin area, and the soles of the feet. Otherwise, just let it be, unless you are dirty from activity! Apply body oil, like coconut, sesame, neem, and Vata herbal, to damp skin. Do not use neem essential oil directly on the skin if it is not in a carrier oil.

- Wash your face once a day with mild soap or cleansing oil. Splash with cool water, but only use a cleanser once a day or every few days if you have very sensitive skin. Do not use a washcloth. Pat dry and apply oils as noted above.

- Avoid excessive air travel, as that is an extremely dry atmosphere. If you must fly, hydrate before, during, and after the flight. Carry your own thermos and refill with warm water as needed. Don't drink alcohol on the plane as it is also dehydrating.

- When traveling, use oil in all of your orifices to create a barrier for moisture loss. Using ghee or sesame seed oil, oil the nasal passages, ears, anus, and vagina. Just place a few drops of oil on your finger and apply every few hours.

- Follow the oral care steps on page 92. The most important ones for dry skin are oil pulling and gargling. When we create an oil barrier to keep moisture in any part of the body, even the cheeks and gums, it will help overall dry skin conditions.

- If you swim, apply oil, like coconut oil, to your entire body, including your scalp, beforehand. Coconut oil protects you from the sun's harmful rays and it will put a barrier between you and the chemicals in the swimming pool.

APOTHECARY

- Apply aloe vera gel to dry skin. Drink 2 to 4 tablespoons (30 to 60 ml) a day of aloe vera liquid.

- Manjistha cleans the blood and liver of toxins, having an especially powerful effect on the complexion. Buy the powder to use as a face mask, and to make tea. Take ½ teaspoon in a mug of hot water twice a day. For a super cleanse, try ½ teaspoon of manjistha and ½ teaspoon of neem powder. Mix with warm water and drink two to three times a day.

- Hibiscus is a natural skin booster. Use the powder to make tea or paste for a face mask. For the tea, take ½ teaspoon in a mug of warm water once or twice a day. To make a paste, add a teaspoon of powder to your palm and keep adding drops of water until a thick paste forms. Hibiscus is also great for the hair and scalp. Add a few tablespoons (7.5 g) of the powder to a cup of water (240 ml) for a hair rinse. There are no contraindications.

- Licorice tea, made from ¼ teaspoon of licorice powder in a mug of water, once or twice a day, will lubricate the tissues in the body, helping you stay hydrated from the inside out.

- Conventional supplements such as vitamin E, vitamin C, vitamin B, and zinc improve dry skin. It's always preferable to eat food containing these nutrients, but in a pinch, the supplements work too.

Ideal Face Wash Routine by Dosha

Vata skin tends to be dry, thin, sensitive, and lacking in elasticity. Pitta and Kapha both have more oil naturally occurring in their skin, but Pitta skin leans toward redness (rosacea, heat rash), while Kapha skin is more cold, clammy, and slightly thicker than the other doshas. Note: Particular oils, herbs, and washes can either calm or irritate. Go slowly.

VATA

Daily: Splash your face with warm water in the morning without cleanser. Pat dry but leave slightly moist. Apply a Vata-calming oil, such as olive, coconut, ghee, or sesame, to a damp face. Alternatively, spray a hydro-mist onto your face or palms and mix with three to five drops of oil. Oil your lips and the inside of your nostrils. Press your palms into your cheeks, forehead, neck, and around and under your nose. Pressing ensures the skin absorbs the oil.

Once or twice a week: Combine 1 tablespoon (20 g) of raw honey with 1 tablespoon (15 g) of triphala powder. Mix with a small amount of warm water. Blend and apply in an even layer to your face and neck. Allow it to dry anywhere from 15 to 30 minutes. Rinse with warm water, pat dry, and apply a thin layer of Vata-calming oils. Or use a banana-egg face mask. This mask is packed with nutrients for your skin. In a blender, blend a ripe banana, an egg yolk, and 1 tablespoon (20 g) of raw honey. Whip and apply to your face and neck for 15 to 30 minutes. Allow it to dry and rinse with warm water.

(continued)

PITTA

Daily: Splash your face and eyes with cool water morning and evening to calm the heat of Pitta. In the morning, after splashing, pat dry and apply Pitta-calming facial oil such as hibiscus, olive, sesame, or ghee to a damp face. Alternatively, spray a hydro-mist onto your face or palms and mix with three to five drops of oil. Oil lips and nostrils, too. In the evening, apply oil to cleanse the face. Use any of the oils above or neem in a carrier oil. Gently massage the oil into your face in a circular motion. Allow it to be absorbed for a minute or two, then take a warm washcloth and gently press it onto the skin to absorb excess oil and any dirt or makeup from the day. For an emotional boost, as well as a skin cooler, pat two to four drops of grapefruit essential oil onto the face and neck, and around the ears.

Once or twice a week: Make a face mask from 1 tablespoon (15 g) of hibiscus powder and 1 tablespoon (15 g) of neem powder. Mix with a small amount of water to make a paste. Apply an even layer to your face and neck. Allow it to dry anywhere from 15 to 30 minutes. Rinse with warm water, pat dry, and apply a thin layer of any Pitta-calming oils. A cooling mask for Pitta, especially beneficial in summer, is an avocado-cucumber mask. Blend a cucumber and the pulp of one avocado. Apply to your face and neck, allow it to dry, then rinse off.

KAPHA

Daily: Kapha rarely has dry skin as they naturally have more oil than the other doshas, but they get more dry as they move more into the later years of life (associated with Vata dosha). If this is the case, follow the guidelines above for Vata. Even if you are not experiencing dry skin, it is always wise to not overwash. A splash of water in the morning, followed by a few drops of sesame seed oil or jojoba oil, with herbs or essential oils like grapefruit, clary sage, or bergamot, reduces oil and sebum production. Using wet palms, press the oil into the skin. In the evening, rinse with a mild soap like a neem or lavender soap, pat dry, and apply oil under the eyes or wherever it's needed.

Once or twice a week: Apply a mask made from 1 tablespoon (15 g) of triphala powder and 1 tablespoon (20 g) of raw honey mixed with warm water to create a paste. Apply an even layer to your face and neck. Allow it to dry anywhere from 15 to 30 minutes. Rinse with warm water, pat dry, and apply a thin layer of a Kapha-calming oil.

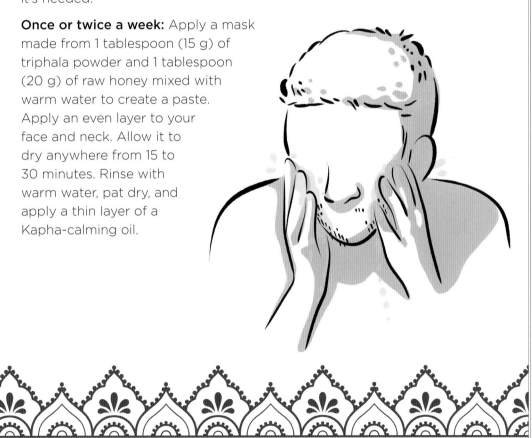

Nourishing Massage

One of the easiest and most enjoyable ways to maintain healthy skin is to do an Ayurvedic massage called abhyanga (page 174), every day if possible.

Vata
- Sesame seed oil or an herbal blend designed to reduce Vata.

Pitta
- Combine coconut and sesame seed oils.

Kapha
- Add some mustard seed oil to sesame seed or sunflower oil for an extra boost.

Warm the oil by running the bottle under hot water.

Stand on a towel or a bath mat you won't mind getting oily.

Put about a quarter-sized amount of oil in your palm and apply the oil to your body, beginning with your scalp, neck, and face and working your way down. Add more oil as needed. Use long, deep strokes and cover your entire body with the oil, moving up and down over the long bones and in a circular motion over your joints, tummy, and hips. Concentrate on areas that may be achy or have pains. Press the oil deep into your skin.

If you have the time, allow the oil to penetrate the skin deeply by leaving it on for 15 to 20 minutes before showering or bathing. If you do not have time for a full-body massage, focus on massaging your joints, head, and feet.

After the massage, shower or bathe to remove most of the excess oil. No need to use soap. Leave a thin layer of oil on the skin to stay moisturized, keep environmental toxins out, and allow the skin's microbiome to flourish.

If applying after bathing, allow the oil to sink into the skin before putting on clothes. You may dab excess oil off with a towel prior to dressing.

Condition: Toenail Fungus

Toenail fungus appears in several ways: thickening of the toenail, yellow or white discolorations, or a foul odor akin to a dirty socks smell. There can be pain, especially in ill-fitting shoes. I am including it here under skin conditions, as it affects not only the nail and the nail bed, but penetrates the epidermis as well. As a yeast infection primarily, this condition is challenging to clear up. Keep up these practices daily as fungus growing on our skin disrupts the entire system. It can take months to eradicate so stay vigilant, and with time, it can be healed.

FOOD

- Reduce sugar. Yeast thrives in that sweet environment. Avoid white sugar completely and eat sweet fruits in moderation. Consume raw honey, especially Manuka honey, as it has extremely nourishing, antibacterial properties. Apply it topically as well.

- Eat only slow-burning complex carbohydrates such as greens, peas, beans, and whole grains.

- Avoid greasy, fast, fried, and processed foods. These will create ama (toxins) in your gut and further the spread of bacteria. A clean diet will help to clean up the fungus.

LIFESTYLE

- Wash your feet every day and be sure to dry them completely, especially the area affected by the fungus.

- As often as possible, keep your toes exposed to the air by wearing sandals or other open-toed shoes.

- If you must wear socks, use only organic materials, such as cotton or hemp, and change frequently so the fungal area stays dry. Avoid all synthetic materials, such as polyester or Lycra, as they trap moisture against the toes. Some sport socks have moisture-wicking material, which may be effective.

- If your shoes are old and dirty, get rid of them. Keep feet and shoes clean and dry.

- Make sure your shoes are the right size. Have some space between the toes and the front of the shoes. Air and space are important in preventing the fungus from growing.

APOTHECARY

- There are many home remedies for toenail fungus. Try each one for about two months. If you don't see any relief in that time, move on to the next one. Fungus is tricky and hard to pin down. Hopefully one of these will work for you!

- Turmeric may help get rid of fungus: First, dust the area with turmeric powder and rub it into the affected area. To make a paste, add ½ teaspoon of turmeric powder to a small amount of water and mix. Apply this once or twice a day. After it dries completely, wash it off and dry the feet thoroughly.

- Tea tree oil is antifungal and reduces signs of infection. In the morning and evening, apply a few drops of oil onto a cotton ball and dab it all around the area. Allow it to dry before putting shoes or socks on.

- Mix 1 teaspoon of olive oil with a few drops of oregano oil, which is antifungal, antibacterial, and antiviral. Other oils to mix with olive oil include lavender, tea tree, calendula, clove, neem, and chamomile. Apply twice a day and allow it to be absorbed before putting on shoes or socks.

- Ayurvedic herbs, triphala and guggulu, pack a huge detoxifying punch. Use ½ teaspoon of each powder and some warm water to make a thick paste. Apply twice a day, allow to dry completely, then wash and dry.

- Create a foot soak with baking soda, apple cider vinegar, and warm water. Use ¼ cup (60 g) of baking soda, 1 cup (235 ml) of apple cider vinegar, and 10 cups (2.4 L) of warm water. Mix these using a bucket or foot soak tub and place your feet in the soak for 30 minutes. Do this once a day until the fungus is gone. Remember to dry your feet completely.

Conditions: Scars, Burns, and Wounds

We all get a few bumps and bruises in our lifetime, but some people suffer serious injuries and accidents that leave their mark on the skin forever. When I was thirteen years old, I fell through a glass door, nearly severing my left arm completely and deeply lacerating my back and legs. After the incredible medical team put me back together and casts and braces came off, I was left with an astonishing array of scars.

While physical recovery was the focus of my healing, I was, of course, consumed by the scars on my skin. At thirteen years old a pimple could throw me for a week, but now I had to deal with over 400 stitches' worth of thick, red, uneven, bumpy, long scars. I was told that after the stitches were removed and the scars began to heal, I could apply shea butter and vitamin E to help further the healing. Over-the-counter options seemed suspicious and even smelly, so shea butter and vitamin E it was, for years. I wish I had known about Ayurveda then, but I'm glad I do now.

This advice is for non-emergencies. If you have a serious accident, cut, or broken bones, seek medical attention immediately. Use the information for healing scars once you are treated and recovering.

If you are hurt, clean the wound immediately with warm water and soap and gently dry. Apply pressure to stop bleeding. After taking the normal steps for a cut, burn, or wound, follow these protocols for healing and scar reduction only. Treat the wound as soon as possible to lessen the chance of a prominent scar.

FOOD

- Eat a balanced diet with carbohydrates, protein, fiber, and fats. You may need more protein while healing.

- Add bone broth into your daily routine while healing. One cup a day of beef or chicken bone broth will deliver collagen and protein, which are both key to wound healing.

- To heal your skin, get more vitamin C through foods such as strawberries, Brussels sprouts, cabbage, cauliflower, broccoli, and citrus fruits. Zinc is also important to wound healing and can be found in pumpkin seeds, peanuts, cashews, almonds, eggs, chocolate, whole milk, meat, shellfish, chickpeas, lentils, and legumes. Omega-3 fatty acids contain antioxidants and retinols, which reduce inflammation and help scars heal faster as well. Eat salmon, anchovies, sardines, and mackerel, which have high omega-3 content.

- Add a teaspoon a day of turmeric into your diet. Sauté it in ghee and add to savory foods or make a hot drink, such as Golden Milk (page 25) with ½ teaspoon of turmeric in 12 ounces (355 ml) of whole milk. Add a pinch of cinnamon, nutmeg, and black pepper, and ½ teaspoon of ghee for better absorption.

LIFESTYLE

- When the wound is healing, expose it to fresh air as soon as possible. The oxygen and air will help to re-establish the microbiome.

- Wear loose clothing over the area. All-natural fibers are best.

- Avoid swimming in chlorinated pools until the wound is completely healed.

- Never use harsh soaps or scrubs on the area. Always pat dry.

- Be sure to get enough sleep. That's 7 to 9 hours for most people. Our bodies heal while we sleep.

APOTHECARY

- Try turmeric. Make a paste from turmeric powder and apply it directly to the wound. Cover with a clean cloth or bandage. Make sure the bleeding has stopped before applying.

- For minor cuts and scrapes, apply tea tree oil directly to the injury—just a drop or two as this is a powerful antiseptic.

- Apply aloe vera gel to wounds with pain or swelling, or a minor burn. Look for one that doesn't have dyes or any other additives.

- Ghee works well for minor burns. Apply a thin layer and leave open to the air.

- Neem oil is an antiseptic and accelerates healing. Applying neem early to an injury will reduce your chances of getting a scar.

- After the wound has begun to heal, gently massage the area two to three times every day with coconut oil.

- The Ayurvedic herb *gotu kola* also is a great healer of scars. Apply as a paste or take as a tea or oral supplement. Gotu kola acts like a steroid to heal the tissues, without the negative side effects. Take one or two tablets a day (60 to 150 mg) while healing. This is not recommended for pregnant women.

- Apply castor oil directly to wounds to increase the lymphocytes around the wound, which will increase healing and reduce scarring.

Case Study

Laura came to me for depression and nearly constant stomachaches. Almost everything she ate gave her cramps, and she never knew when she would need to use the bathroom. She hated eating out and hesitated to have people over to her house. This exacerbated her depression and grief at losing a loved one a few years prior.

Why am I including this scenario under the topic of skin? Because it was revealed during our intake session that Laura had been taking antibiotics for more than twenty years. Daily. For more than twenty years. I nearly fell off my chair. A doctor had prescribed her the drug for adult-onset acne and Laura, now forty-five years old, was afraid that if she stopped the acne would return.

Besides the fact that I simply could not believe a doctor would continue this for two decades, it all made sense to me. Every symptom Laura had was related to antibiotic use. Antibiotics work for acne because they wipe out bacteria in the system, including bacteria that causes acne. Out with the bad is out with the good. Her body was struggling daily to replenish the gut and skin microbiome but was losing out to the daily antibiotic. Not only did her doctor not warn her about the possible resistance to future antibiotic use, but he did not discuss probiotic benefits or even skin care.

The result was decades of diarrhea, gut issues, lethargy, and indecisiveness. She stayed too long in situations that were not healthy for her and was unable to move forward in life. The depression was likely caused by the compromised microbiome in the gut, where our "happy" hormones are produced, like serotonin, dopamine, and oxytocin. Not to mention the long-term damage to her liver, where the antibiotics were processed. I call the liver the washing machine of the body. If it is constantly under attack, we suffer because the liver cannot properly process everything else that enters the machine— our body.

Working with her doctor, we devised a plan for Laura to stop taking the antibiotics and begin a regimen to detox her gut and liver. She took the powerful Ayurvedic herb manjistha, which has amazing healing properties for both the skin and liver. This blood purifier detoxes and supports blood circulation to create a clear, healthy complexion. Other powerful herbs she took included neem and bhumyamalaki, both known to clean the blood and liver, and provide general detox, completing the supplement package to heal her skin and gut. She stayed on these herbs for six weeks.

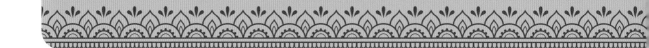

After the Ayurvedic herbs cleansed the liver and gut, Laura took a powerful probiotic called Trenev Trio to repopulate her gut with trillions of live bacteria. Her symptoms really turned around, and she seemed like a new woman. Additionally, instructions were given (and followed) to leave her skin alone! The temptation to overwash is great, but the skin is happiest with the occasional use of gentle oils and cleansers to rebuild its microbiome of healthy bacteria, enabling it to fight off environmental toxins. Using tender methods of cleaning the skin, including oils mixed with hydrosol waters, patting dry, and pressing the oil/water mixture into the skin once a day, we were able to find the right balance.

For Laura, the process was to wash her face once a day with neem and aloe soap. Just a small amount of soap rubbed into the face and neck, then splashed with water. No washcloth, no scrubbing. Pat dry with a fully organic cotton towel and apply two to three drops of neem oil with sandalwood hydrosol spray to the face and neck. Pat and press the oil/water mix gently into the skin.

Laura's gut issues took about three months to resolve, which is amazing after twenty years of abuse, but the body is resilient and, given time, herbs, and proper care, it will bounce back. Her depression lifted as she incorporated plant-based foods into her diet and reduced dairy, unhealthy oils, and non-organic wheat. As the gut improved, circulation and detoxification improved and, on top of everything else, Laura's skin looked beautiful.

There was no need to continue any of the herbal supplements or the probiotic after the symptoms cleared up. Laura was able to maintain a healthy balance by eating prebiotic and probiotic foods, continuing a gentle skin-care routine, and following a regimen for her dosha.

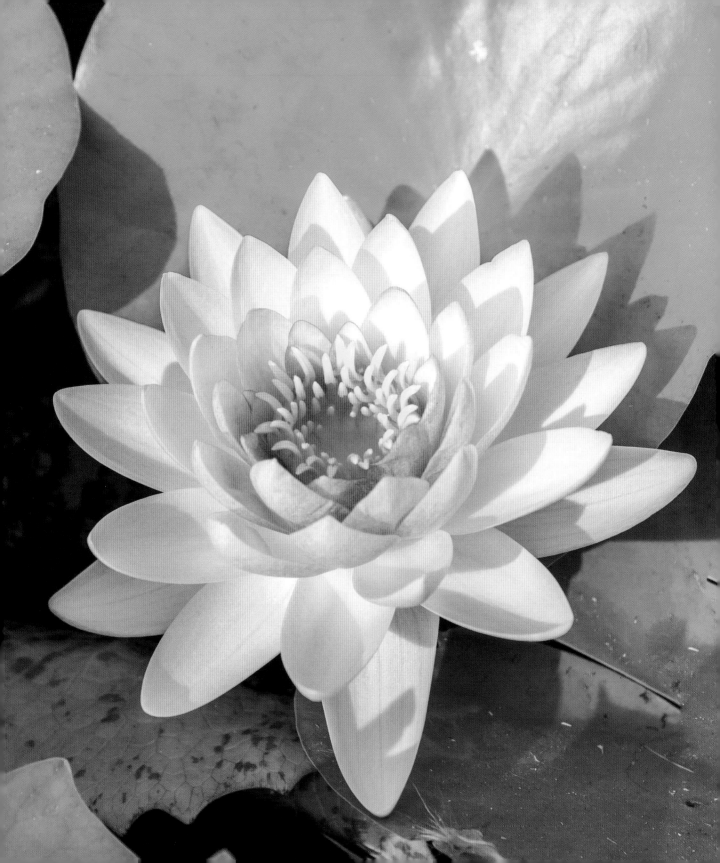

6

Reproductive System: Healthy for Life

The reproductive organs and tissues (*shukra* and *artava dhatu*) are important at every stage of life. Libido, fertility, menstruation, dryness, menopause, and andropause are managed by paying attention to this dhatu. These tissues grow from birth to puberty and fertility, becoming robust. After the age of thirty-five to forty, the primary use for these organs (reproduction) fades. In Ayurveda, we call the juice or nectar that is secreted in stages of youth and good health *ojas*. As we age, ojas depletes. Less nourishment is absorbed in this dhatu due to the natural process of hormonal depletion. With care and attention, we can feed and nourish the organs to ensure that this area stays robust, moist, and healthy—able to both receive nutrients and eliminate waste until the end of life.

Ayurveda and Reproductive Health

Our reproductive organs are the center of the sacral chakra (*swadhistana*). This chakra is the center of creativity, sexuality, intimacy, and emotional intelligence. The sacral chakra is watery, allowing for a healthy flow of nutrients and emotions. It is below the navel and above the pelvic bones. Located just below it is the root chakra (*mulhadarah*), which keeps us grounded, safe, stable, and secure.

These two chakras work with the other five chakras, but it's these two that most directly relate to sex. While the seven main chakras (root, sacral, solar plexus, heart, throat, third eye, and crown) ideally will be balanced for a healthy sex life and life in general, we'll look at how to support and increase the qualities we need in the sacral area.

Grounding, stability, fluidity, creativity, and movement define this area. If the organs and tissues get dry, blocked, and stagnant, it will slow us down in many facets of our life. The importance of staying pliable affects us on every level. We need good flow in urination and menstruation. We need sexual energy and desire, the ability to dream and create. Additionally, the next chakra up is the solar plexus, which is a center of power. That energy can give us a boost to create and flow in all areas of our lives. It's all connected here.

FOOD: FEEDING THE LOWER CHAKRAS

- Focus on foods that align with the colors of the first three chakras. Red for the root, orange for the sacral, and yellow for the solar plexus. Red, orange, and yellow bell peppers; apples, oranges, and bananas; carrots, red beets, and golden beets; orange roughy fish and salmon; ghee, turmeric, and saffron.

- Hydrate with nourishing drinks, warm smoothies, and soups. Combine densely nutritive, grounding foods like dates, almonds, and oats (or oat milk) to make an ojas-rejuvenating smoothie. Throw a handful of oats, bulgur wheat, or farro (an ancient grain) into a pot of soup for an extra ojas-building boost. Use ghee abundantly.

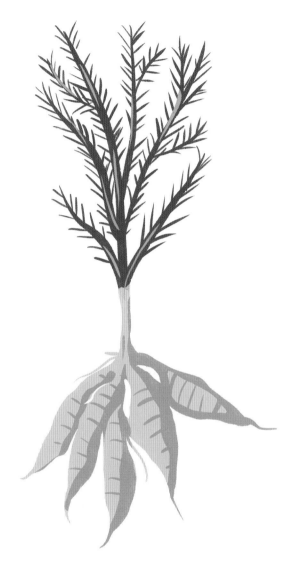

LIFESTYLE: SASSY AND SEXY

- Lean in to your desires and dreams. Ignore pressure to conform to society's views of what an older person should look like. Dress however you want. Do your hair in your favorite styles.

- Dress to avoid harsh elements on sensitive skin. Wear a scarf to protect your neck from sun and wind damage. Cover your arms from the harsh sun.

- Wear comfortable shoes and clothing. (I did not say "sensible"!) Feet can widen as we age and toes can spread. Wear shoes with a wide toe box and avoid anything that restricts movement.

APOTHECARY: ROBUST AT ANY AGE

Shatavari. This is one of Ayurveda's wonder herbs that repairs many issues. In addition to overall feminine health, it is appropriate for all genders to improve libido and sexual function, increase vaginal lubrication in women, enhance sensitivity of the nipples, and promote feelings of love and devotion. Note that shatavari boosts fertility. Take one to two tablets a day before food. Shatavari comes from the asparagus root, so if you have an allergy to asparagus avoid this supplement.

- Ashwagandha. In Sanskrit *ashwagandha* means "strength of a horse." It is an adaptogen that responds to what the nervous system needs, promoting healthy sleep as well as maintaining a relaxed energy, allowing the body to heal and function at the highest level. The aging process is supported by this herb, as it rejuvenates and promotes strong muscles, joint health, and bone density. Take two tablets before bed for four weeks and notice if your sleep improves. If so, continue to take in the evening. Alternatively, you can take two during the day, with food, to maintain good health and energy. Take for as long as needed.

Condition: Low Libido

Many of us, as we navigate puberty, cannot imagine a day when we might not be very interested in sex. But alas, it happens. Stress, age, negative or traumatic experiences, poor nutrition, and lifestyle choices might erode our natural sexual desires. Ayurveda wants to ensure that we have a healthy libido at every stage of life as this area is an important energy center.

Ayurveda says that sex with someone you love will enhance your libido, but, conversely, sex with someone you do not love will deplete you. If desire is suppressed, emotional and physical issues may arise. Sex with someone you love reflects the qualities of chakras that help keep you feeling intimate, safe, and secure as well as in touch with your sexuality.

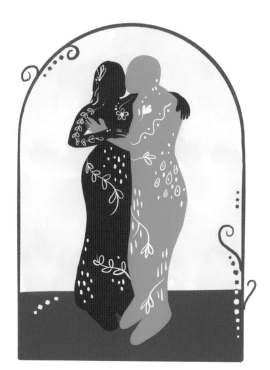

There are ways to increase your libido, but remember to eat well, sleep well, move your body, and be mindful of all the healthy practices we have talked about. These remedies are aphrodisiacs. Interestingly, the Sanskrit word for male aphrodisiacs is *Vajikarana*, which literally means "horse power."

FOOD

- Watch your weight. Overeating and undereating both deplete your sexual energy. Strive for a balanced diet that is appropriate for your dosha. Avoid fried, overly fatty, and processed food.

- If you drink alcohol, choose one to two servings of beer and wine. Avoid spirits; they will ultimately depress sexual desire.

- Food that increases blood flow aids in sexual desire and function. Those foods include oysters; lobster, crab, and seafood high in zinc; antioxidant- and nitrate-rich foods such as beets, celery, spinach, and arugula; nuts and seeds; fresh fruit; cocoa and green tea. The allicin in garlic is an enhancer, but be sure to brush your teeth after! These foods are heart healthy and increase blood flow.

LIFESTYLE

- Sleep is essential to all aspects of life, libido included. If you do not sleep well at night and wake feeling unrested, the rest of your physical, emotional, and spiritual functions will be limited.

- Connect with your partner on a deeper level by meditating, listening to guided meditations, and even listening to podcasts dealing with relationships, sexuality, and erotica. By participating in these activities together, you are creating trust, which is key to a robust libido. You may also consider seeing a counselor, couple's therapist, or sex therapist to help you uncover issues and create deeper bonds.

- All genders should see a doctor to rule out low libido as an indicator of serious issues, and be certain to get enough physical exercise to maintain healthy airways, blood flow, and stamina.

APOTHECARY

Please note: These recommendations are widely available on the internet, but should be taken under the guidance of an Ayurvedic, Traditional Chinese Medicine, functional medicine, or homeopathic practitioner or naturopath.

- Traditional Ayurveda recommends an herb called *safed musli*, which has been called an alternative to Viagra. However, in addition to increasing blood flow and other physical components, safed musli acts on the mind as an aphrodisiac.

Ojas–Replenishing Treat

While sex can be amazing it also can sap energy and leave us feeling drained. In Ayurveda, when we expel a huge amount of energy, we look to nourish and replenish ourselves. Ojas is that essence of life, and when we feel drained, even from a good thing, it means we have used up a good amount of ojas. Don't despair! Here is a treat that restores ojas, increases energy, and is delicious. This recipe serves two, but feel free to increase it for more.

Serves 2

- 6 large Medjool dates, pitted
- 6 almonds, soaked in hot water, and peeled
- 1 tablespoon (15 g) ghee
- ½ orange, juiced

Open the dates and insert one almond into each. In a frying pan, melt the ghee over medium heat. Place the dates in the pan, turning once or twice to coat them in ghee. Add the orange juice to the ghee and dates and stir gently so as not to knock the almonds out of the dates. Sauté the dates in the mixture for about 3 to 5 minutes, or until hot. Remove and place on a plate. Allow them to cool just a bit and enjoy!

- *Gokshura* comes from a small shrub and is found worldwide. It will increase lubrication, arousal, and desire and can be used by all genders. In powder form, add ¼ to ½ teaspoon to warm water and drink once a day before food. Do not take if you are pregnant or nursing.

- *Brahmi* is known as a brain tonic, supporting memory and the nervous system. As such, it supports a healthy libido. One exceptional by-product is that it is great for your hair, too! Another is its ability to promote awareness and alertness that help you to be mindful of you and your partner, allowing for more trust and openness. Take one to two tablets a day after food.

- While food, herbs, and supplements nudge you in the right direction, aphrodisiacs are not the final solution. Take a deeper look into your personal relationships and note where you might improve your connections. Be better equipped to make good choices and live a stress-free life by staying healthy mentally and physically. This will boost your sexual desire too.

Condition: Infertility

I could write an entire book on Ayurveda and fertility, and several people have. It's such a vast and important topic as so many struggle with the ability to get pregnant. We live in a world where people postpone trying to get pregnant until they are past the age of their highest fertility. In addition to that, stress, the environment, poor food and drink choices, and hormones in the foods we eat all play a role.

If you are having trouble getting pregnant, I suggest you visit an Ayurvedic practitioner who specializes in this area. There are so many reasons for the condition, and individual care is necessary to help you be successful. On the journey to motherhood, please consider these steps.

FOOD

- Keep the tissues nourished by eating a diet rich in good fats such as ghee, avocado and olive oil, nuts, and seeds. Eat foods high in folic acid such as beans, peas, lentils, and eggs, and low in mercury, like some types of fish. High-fiber foods are key, so eat veggies, oatmeal, and whole grains.

- Avoid processed meats, alcohol, and simple carbohydrates such as syrups, candy, and sweeteners.

LIFESTYLE

- Being overweight or underweight negatively impacts your chances of getting pregnant. Try to maintain a weight that is reasonable for your frame. This means thin for Vata, medium build for Pitta, and slightly larger/curvier for Kapha.

- Meditate for stress reduction and use visualization to see yourself as fertile, becoming pregnant, and birthing a healthy baby.

- Make sure you get the right amount of sleep, which is usually between 7 and 9 hours a night. Sleeping at the appropriate times is important for the highest level of body function. Get to sleep by 10 p.m.

- Relax. Have date nights. Talk about all the possible ways of having a baby, including IVF, surrogates, and adoption. Know that there are options. Enjoy the company of your partner, if you have one, or good friends and family who do not put pressure on you. Try not to put pressure on yourself.

APOTHECARY

- Herbs that support the female reproductive tissues include shatavari, brahmi, vidari kanda, and guduchi. These should be taken under the advice of a consultant who is familiar with any other medication you are taking.

- Do abhyanga self-massage (page 174) daily with sesame or almond oil. Apply the oil to the entire body and allow it to seep into the skin for 20 minutes, then rinse off.

Condition: Vaginal Dryness

This painful condition usually occurs during menopause as estrogen decreases and the vaginal tissues thin. It may also occur due to medication, medical conditions, or extreme Vata imbalance. A dry, thin vaginal wall makes it very uncomfortable to have intercourse, exercise, and even urinate. Diet, oils, supplements, and some lifestyle changes will help you find relief.

FOOD

- Follow all the food rules for menopause. Avoid becoming dehydrated by sipping warm or room temperature water throughout the day. Incorporating watery foods, such as zucchini, watermelon, chia seeds, and flaxseed, in your diet helps.

- Eat a Vata-pacifying diet that includes nutrient-dense foods such as dairy, nuts, nut butters, healthy grains, some meat, avocados, and sweet juicy fruits.

LIFESTYLE

- Wear loose, 100 percent organic cotton underwear. Avoid tight pants and jeans. Allow for natural air flow.

- Use wet wipes after urinating rather than toilet paper, and pat rather than rubbing. Do not use soap on or around your vagina. Just rinse the area with warm water. Harsh chemicals will hurt and increase dryness.

- Be sure to use a natural laundry detergent and avoid all perfume, powder, and lotions in the vaginal area.

- Avoid tampons and notice if certain condoms make the condition worse. Remember to talk to your partner about your condition and let them know what hurts and what feels better. Taking your time during foreplay or using coconut oil or ghee increases lubrication.

- Quit smoking ASAP.

APOTHECARY

- Our favorite female rejuvenative, shatavari, is a lifesaver. It naturally increases lubrication. Take two tablets before food, once or twice a day.

- Specific oils as topical applications help each dosha. Use organic oils only, such as sesame, coconut and ghee. Apply to the labia area as needed. Eat more ghee, too.

- Drink 2 ounces (60 ml) of aloe vera juice in the morning on an empty stomach daily.

- Drink licorice tea or take licorice powder (½ teaspoon) once a day before food. Do not take licorice if you are pregnant.

- Perform abhyanga massage (page 174) every day. This external oiling of the body penetrates through the tissues and will help to ease all dryness in the body.

Condition: Vaginal Yeast (Candida) Infections

Yeast, or *Candida*, lives in our bodies, usually in harmony with the other bacteria until something comes along and disrupts it. Infections take root when one has sluggish, low digestive fire, called *manda agni* in Sanskrit. The result is ama, meaning undigested food that will eventually become a toxic, fermenting mess in the gut, disrupting the microbiome, spreading out to the rest of our tissues, and creating a host of unhealthy microbial activity. This leads to overgrowth of yeast, which may show up in the digestive track, the blood, eventually into skin folds, the anus, and the vagina. Other causes are antibiotic use, stress, poor sleep, high sugar intake, and obesity.

The white, sticky qualities of a yeast infection point to a Kaphic imbalance. Kapha is heavy, unctuous, sticky, wet, and cold, just like yeast. Some yeast infections look more Pitta in nature with a thinner, milky discharge and slightly yellow. This means that some of both Kapha and Pitta food guidelines must be followed.

One must be vigilant in following the protocols as yeast infections are notoriously difficult to eradicate. Conventional medicine is effective, but the chemicals used to clear up the *Candida* may have negative side effects, such as killing all the *Candida*, rather than re-creating the balance that once existed. If you have a stubborn yeast infection that will not clear up, despite having followed the treatments, a combination of Western and Eastern may be needed.

If you have had one, you know that yeast infections cause burning when urinating, a foul odor, unbearable itching, inflammation, irritation, and/or a thick white or thinner, yellow discharge. The discomfort might last for weeks as one searches for a cause (often diagnosed as vaginitis) and a cure. Nearly 75 percent of women will have a vaginal yeast infection in her lifetime. Mine came when using the "sponge" for birth control in the 80s. Those spermicidal chemicals did not suit my body, and I found myself with a terribly difficult-to-cure reaction: a raging yeast infection. I applied yogurt, sat in apple cider vinegar baths, and probably did a few other home cures.

In the end, though, I remember taking Diflucan (fluconazole) by mouth. I'm sure my gut suffered, but back then I didn't know how to support myself while taking a drug that wipes out fungus. There are legions of home remedies, but sometimes the pain and discomfort win out and we turn to an over-the-counter cream or a prescription drug. I share these details with you hoping that if you need to take a Western drug, you can follow the guidelines here to help rebuild your gut microbiome and get you back into balance.

FOOD

- Strictly follow a diet containing no sugar, including fructose, honey, jaggery, coconut palm sugar, maple syrup, or date syrup. This means no fresh or dried fruits or fruit juices. *Candida* thrives in sugar, so to wipe it out, cut off its food source.

- Stay away from fermented foods, yeasted breads, and crackers (anything with yeast in the ingredients). Kapha-genic (food that increases Kapha) foods should be avoided, including dairy, wheat, and sugar. Avoid mushrooms, vinegar, pasta, hard cheese, peanuts, and baked goods. Gluten-free is best. Avoid heavy, oily foods, fried food, and fast food.

- Eat lots of dark, leafy greens and nonstarchy vegetables such as broccoli, cauliflower, kale, romaine lettuce, and green, yellow, and red peppers. Avoid squash, corn, potatoes, yams, cassava, parsnips, and sugary veggies such as beets and carrots.

- Use ghee, sesame seed oil, or olive oil. Be sure to include these spices in your diet: turmeric, ginger, cinnamon, cardamom, cumin, and hing (asafoetida).

- Eliminate caffeine as it is a diuretic. Drink hot water with lemon or lime and herbal teas. Try to stay consistently hydrated as that will help to detox the body. Avoid drinking alcohol as it converts to pure sugar. A good substitute for a sparkling drink is kombucha or KeVita, which is a water-based kefir drink.

LIFESTYLE

- Wear loose organic cotton or other breathable material for underwear. Don't wear tight pants (including yoga pants) or leggings, tights, or stockings. The vaginal area must be allowed to breathe and air out.

- Get 7 to 9 hours of sleep a night; go to sleep no later than 10 p.m. Sound sleep is healing for the entire system. Sleep on organic cotton sheets and go without underwear.

- Relax and rest. The body has been invaded by an overgrowth of fungus. You may feel depleted, so give in to it and take it easy. Avoid naps, but if you feel sleepy in the daytime, try resting sitting up for 10 to 15 minutes.

- Don't have sex until the infection is completely cleared. Yeast infections are not contagious, but sex will further irritate the area and make it uncomfortable or painful.

APOTHECARY

- Take a good probiotic that contains live bacteria, including *Lactobacillus acidophilus* and *Bifidobacteria bifidum*.

- Wash with triphala powder for Kaphic, thick white, smelly discharge. Take 1 tablespoon (15 g) of triphala powder in 2 cups (475 ml) of warm water. Allow the triphala to steep for 10 minutes. Soak a washcloth in the mix and apply to the vagina, gently allowing the solution to cover the entire area. Keep bathing in the mix for 5 minutes. Neem or licorice powder can be substituted for triphala.

- Use a mix of diluted tea tree oil with honey. In a small bowl add 1 cup (235 ml) of warm water to three to five drops of tea tree oil and 1 tablespoon (20 g) of raw honey. Use Manuka honey if you have it. Apply to the vagina with a cloth and allow it to penetrate the area for 10 to 15 minutes, then rinse off and pat dry.

- Wipe clean with a cool washcloth. Some women prefer a cool washcloth. If the above application is not comfortable, allow the compounds to cool off, or add cool water.

- Some people swear by full-fat, organic plain yogurt. Apply liberally to the entire vaginal area. Eat a small bowl every day too. Make sure the yogurt has live bacteria.

- For itchy, inflamed infections, use aloe vera gel or coconut oil topically several times a day. Allow the gel or oil to dry completely before getting dressed.

- Apply apple cider vinegar with a washcloth or cotton balls. Leave it on for 5 minutes and wipe off, twice a day. Drink 1 teaspoon ACV in warm water once a day, on an empty stomach.

Condition: Andropause

Over the years, my male clients have come in with a host of symptoms with seemingly "no cause" to pin them to. It's just growing old, some will say. When I point out that they are of the age of andropause, most of them have never heard of the term. Some have heard about "male menopause," but andropause remains elusive and not well understood by many.

Andras in Greek means "human male," and *pause* in Greek means "cessation"; andropause is defined as a syndrome associated with a decrease in sexual satisfaction or a decline in a feeling of general well-being with low levels of testosterone in older men. With aging, hormone levels change to accommodate what is required of the body. As men and women grow older and pass the age of fertility, when robust hormone production to procreate is no longer needed, fewer hormones are produced, causing a host of issues.

As we live longer, we more acutely notice the changes, and some will go to extraordinary lengths to boost hormone production and try to stay youthful longer. Our bodies and minds have innate systems that keep us healthy and vital at each stage of life, but we sometimes fight against it, desiring to feel like we did at twenty-five when we are sixty-five.

Ayurveda is a beautiful system that allows us to age gracefully and naturally while protecting the tissues, keeping them robust and functioning as they were meant to be. We may want to fight against this with hormone injections and supplements, but ultimately, the body will win. Appreciate the wisdom of the body and allow nature to do its job. Appreciate all the stages of life, embrace changes, and work with them rather than against them. I am a big believer in flowing downstream instead of struggling to swim upstream against the tide. If we follow the guidelines for healthy eating, moving, and sleeping, we are flowing.

FOOD

- Eat Vata-pacifying food such as milk, ghee, eggs, poultry, fresh fruits, nuts, grains, greens, and lots of cooked vegetables. Reduce red meat consumption and eat more fish. If you are overweight, consume a bit less of these foods.

- If you do not suffer from Pitta issues, such as heartburn, increase intake of foods and fruits high in lycopene and vitamin C, such as tomatoes, cherries, melons, oranges, and citrus.

- Reduce alcohol intake, excessive sugar, and all processed foods. Stay hydrated to keep the tissues robust. Sip water or herbal tea throughout the day or drink kombucha or KeVita (a water-based kefir drink).

LIFESTYLE

- Create a daily routine and try to stick to it: Sleep and consume meals on a regular schedule. Exercise at the same time of day. This will help your body regulate to the hormonal changes.

- Reduce stress by not pushing yourself so hard to perform in the areas of sex and exercise. Strenuous activity of any kind creates imbalances in mind and body. Try not to go to extremes, such as running in the heat of day or staying out late and getting up too early.

- Do not suppress natural urges, including belching, flatulence, coughing, bowel movements, urination, sneezing, yawning, sleeping, crying, orgasm, hunger, and thirst. Allow your body to express itself naturally. Holding in natural urges increases toxins in the mind and body. We should follow this rule at every age.

- Watch your weight. Being overweight or severely underweight will negatively affect your hormonal balance and other bodily functions. Be aware of any changes and adjust your lifestyle to stay at a steady and healthy weight.

- Muscle mass decreases as testosterone decreases. Stay on top of this by working out with weights and aerobics and stretching. Yoga plus strength training is a great combination to stay strong and flexible.

- Don't smoke.

APOTHECARY

- Daily self-massage on the joints with Vata-reducing oil will keep the tissues nourished and flexible while enabling the body to detox properly. Try to do a whole-body massage a few times a week and rinse off the excess oil after it has been on the body for 20 minutes. See page 174 for details.

- It is just as important for men to maintain a healthy reproductive system as it is for women. For healthy prostate, urine flow, and aphrodisiac effects, try the Ayurvedic herbs ashwagandha, gokshura, amalaki, guggulu, licorice, and vidari kanda. See an Ayurvedic practitioner for more precise dosing for your unique condition.

Condition: Menopause and Hot Flashes

Menopause is a natural transition that all women, if they have a uterus and live long enough, will pass through. I say pass through because you *will* get through it! With a few helpful steps along the way, you may find that you come out happier, stronger, and wiser on the other side.

Menopause is when a woman ceases to have her menstrual period, usually recognized as full-on menopause when there has been no menstrual bleeding for one year. The hormones progesterone and estrogen drop around the age of thirty-five, when most women enter perimenopause, which is the time before the complete cessation of periods as most of the eggs a woman is born with have been depleted. Women's sex hormones decrease as they enter the stage when the eggs are no longer needed to create babies. Don't despair. It's not all lost, and you can rebuild in a different way.

Some women are relieved to be over the fertile stage of life, but many desire to remain sexually active, which supports healthy tissues, moist skin, strong bones, heart health, and emotional satisfaction. A robust reproductive system is necessary to keep women from "drying out" and "shriveling up." Harsh words, I know, but through the actions in this section, you can stave that off and thrive.

Women still can create estrogen even after menopause; it's just less than was needed when fertile. The less stress in your life, the more tissue-nourishing hormones stay in the inventory. Stress depletes in every way, busting the adrenals and producing excess cortisol (these are not good things) and using up precious estrogen and progesterone. By relaxing and chilling out, your sex drive will increase, hot flashes may be lessened, and you'll support more youthful, nourished cells in your entire body.

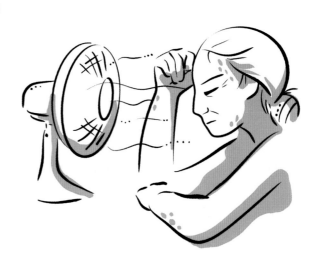

Remember that it is never too early to begin building a foundation for a smooth menopause. By following the guidelines for healthy eating, stress reduction, and exercise, expect your transition from fertile to perimenopause to menopause and post-menopausal to be easier. Don't wait until you are in the throes of hot-flash city to make changes—lay the groundwork now.

It is at the end of the Pitta stage of life and the onset of the Vata stage of life that we find menopause. Perhaps hot flashes are the dying gasps of flames licking at the tissues, searching for depleted hormones, angry and feeling deprived. The winds of Vata fan the embers, increasing heat and hot flashes, as the tissues lose hydration and lubrication.

Some major concerns for women in their menopausal and post-menopausal years are vaginal dryness, low libido, and hormonal fluctuations that cause hot flashes, night sweats, and uncharacteristic behavior—such as emotional hot flashes. Menopause marks a moment in a woman's life where she is given permission to stop looking outward, stop taking care of everyone else, and begin an inward gaze to put her own needs first and take the time to investigate what, exactly, those needs and desires are. Take a look at these remedies and see which ones suit your needs and fit your lifestyle.

Doshic Stages of Life

In Ayurveda, we regard the stages of life according to the doshas—the mind/body constitutions. We are born into a Kaphic stage of life—Kapha comprises the elements of earth and water. As we grow and enter puberty, we begin the Pitta time of life. Pitta is fire and water. We go through school and college or choose a career or lifestyle—headstrong and plowing through the world as if we know best! We may have children or choose not to, move to new places, take on challenges, and make lifestyle decisions that may or may not be best for us.

In the mid-fifties and sixties, we enter the Vata stage of life. Vata has a lot of movement, space, and air, which allows for great expansion of the mind and the ability to share wisdom gathered over the years. The elements of Vata stoke creativity and a sense of "I don't care what anyone else thinks of me. I am living my life on my terms."

FOOD

- Eat estrogenic, supportive foods that are rich in phytoestrogens. Spice your foods with cumin, fennel, hing, turmeric, and coriander to aid digestion. Increase consumption of tofu, tempeh, edamame, miso, flaxseeds, chickpeas, lentils, oats, barley, rice, wheat bran, rye, quinoa, garlic, berries, peaches, yams, dried fruit, and cruciferous veggies. Eating large amounts of soy (more than 16 ounces [450 g] a day) has been linked to an increase in breast cancer, but moderate amounts, 4 to 8 ounces (113 to 225 g) a day, have proven to be beneficial.

- Focus your diet on easy-to-digest foods. These create less heat and improve absorption of liquids, increasing your juiciness! Avoid raw, cold, processed foods. Eat simple meals with just a few ingredients.

- Shift your diet to Pitta-reducing and Vata-increasing foods. This means avoiding acidic, hot, spicy foods. Lean more toward warm, cooked, lightly spiced foods. Choose white basmati rice over brown. Add ghee (a teaspoon for Kapha, more for Vata and Pitta) to just about everything. No refined sugars, but naturally sweet, juicy foods and fruits are good.

- Stay hydrated. This is so important to stave off dryness in the body, internally and externally. Drink water. For good measure, drink half your body weight in ounces.

- For tea, drink 1 to 3 cups a day. Try CCF tea (page 38). Or drink peppermint and spearmint tea or water with a squeeze of lime or with a splash of apple cider vinegar or any of the amazing vinegars on the market. Avoid alcohol, please! Nothing good comes from it during menopause. (Believe me. I tried.) Avoid caffeine too—sorry! If you cannot avoid it completely, at least reduce consumption.

- Eat to detox. Menstruation is one of nature's ways to release toxins from the body. Shedding blood releases excess Pitta, so without that function, find other ways to do it. Eating more bitter and astringent foods like dandelion greens, radicchio, kale, spinach, or cruciferous vegetables (lightly cooked for easy digestion) will support detoxification as well as deeply nourish your body. Use more cilantro and parsley and eat more fiber.

Hot Flash Soother Smoothie

This recipe contains foods that are proven to reduce hot flashes and lessen other symptoms of menopause. Avocado is rich in nutrients and oils to combat dryness. Tofu, with its phytoestrogen, replaces estrogen lost to hormonal changes. Blueberries have flavonoids and vitamins for your brain to alleviate brain fog. Coconut milk is cooling to reduce heat in the body. Flaxseeds and raw honey pack a punch of nutrients. Make enough to drink twice a day. Experiment with plant-based milks to see what works best for you.

Makes 1 to 2 servings

- 1 ripe avocado, skinned and pit removed
- ½ cup (75 g) fresh or frozen blueberries (or any berries)
- ½ block (6 ounces, or 170 g) silken tofu
- 1 teaspoon raw flaxseeds
- 1 tablespoon (20 g) raw honey
- 1 cup (235 ml) coconut milk
- Extra water, if needed

Add all the ingredients to a blender. Blend and split into two servings if you'd like, or drink the entire amount. Enjoy on an empty stomach and don't eat again until you are hungry.

NOTE

If you are lacking fiber in your diet, stir in a tablespoon of psyllium husk (5 g) just before drinking.

- Reduce pungent, spicy foods and totally avoid processed foods, fried food, and food made with unhealthy oils. Eat healthy, nutrient-dense foods, such as sweet fruits, berries, avocados, dates, figs, nuts, seeds, ghee, and olive oil, to increase ojas, which is the essence of life that flows through the body. Look for foods naturally high in calcium, such as bone broth, cottage cheese, and sesame seeds, for bone health. Include choices from bitter and astringent foods (think leafy greens) in every meal.

LIFESTYLE

- Good sleep habits will lessen foggy brain and hot flashes. Get outside as much as possible as nature fosters balance and increases awareness. Walk or jog just enough to get your heart rate and breathing up—about 20 to 30 minutes. Breathe in and out through your nose to increase nitric oxide, which will boost your immune system and clear the cobwebs. Studies show that mouth breathing increases stress and anxiety and a host of dental issues as well.

- Nadi shodhana, or alternate nostril breathing (page 175), reduces hot flashes and slows the mind down. It is crucial for finding balance and peace, especially when mental flare-ups, mood swings, and intense irritability increase when sleep decreases.

- Avoid weight gain but don't make yourself crazy. As hormones find a new level, you may gain a few pounds and cholesterol may increase and then stabilize. Keep up the good habits listed here and be kind to yourself. Two- to three-day seasonal cleanses using the Ayurvedic vegetarian stew called kitchari (page 114) or occasional juice fasts are beneficial, as is eating two to three meals a day and no snacking. Use a juicer only in spring and summer, just a few days a week, as juice contains a lot of sugar and is low in fiber (even though it is high in vitamins and minerals). Avoid juicing in the winter as we need more fiber to keep the body warm.

- Use a wet wipe and pat the vagina to dry after urinating, if you have dryness. Some of my clients have reported great success applying ghee or organic sesame seed oil to the labia throughout the day. Use lubricants to help with intercourse as well.

- Make peace with your past through meditation. Let go of old resentments, anger, and victimhood. These emotions are only damaging you. Through loving-kindness or Metta meditation, make amends with yourself and others. Send love, happiness, safety, and good health to yourself, to your loved ones, to strangers, and to those you have difficulty with. Repeat the phrases "May you be healthy. May you be happy. May you be safe. May you be loved" to all those on the list—and mean it.

APOTHECARY

- Banyan Botanicals formulates some of the best Ayurvedic treatments. Women's Natural Transition and Women's Support are two I highly recommend for keeping the reproductive organs nourished. The herbs in the formulas include shatavari, vidari kanda, ashwagandha, vetiver, brahmi, and others that smooth out menopausal issues as well as deeply replenish and detoxify the tissues. Take two tablets about a half hour before meals, two or three times a day. Do not take shatavari if you are allergic to asparagus, as it comes from the root. (*Shatavari*, by the way, translates as "she who has 100 husbands"!)

- Valerian root, chamomile, and ashwagandha all calm the mind and promote good sleep. Banyan Botanicals' I Sleep Soundly compound will help you do just that. Don't take ashwagandha if you are pregnant.

- Use Bhringaraj oil for a scalp and foot massage before bed. This incredibly powerful oil cools and calms the entire nervous system, promoting peaceful rest. Another benefit is that this oil is known for supporting hair growth and keeping your locks lustrous.

- Do abhyanga, a full-body massage, every day (see page 174). Use a Vata-reducing herbal oil, such as sesame, and apply oil to your limbs in long, slow, deep strokes and in a circular motion around your joints, torso, lower back—everywhere you can reach. Face, neck, ears. Soles of the feet, around your toes and ankles. Allow the oil to penetrate your skin deeply for 20 minutes, then rinse off—or not. Whatever feels best for you!

Case Study

The menopause story I know best is one I am deeply familiar with. It is my own. My periods began when I was twelve years old at summer camp in Asheville, North Carolina, USA, in 1975. Ironically, synchronistically, or magically, my last period was in Asheville in February 2015, where I was attending a booksellers' conference. Of course, I did not know that was going to be my last period until a year later—officially in menopause.

Those final twelve months were sometimes scary as I could have still been fertile, but the odds of getting pregnant were around 1 percent. I had so far avoided having children; I love kids but chose not to have any. Having married at forty-seven, I figured the pressure was off. But I still bought pregnancy test kits and kept them in the bathroom cabinet, testing myself every month—truly petrified I would be one of those few women pregnant in her fifties.

Thankfully that didn't happen. But this is a reality for some women who think they are off the hook (read *Hot Flashes Warm Bottles* by Nancy London if you don't believe me!). Other changes occurred. Emotional rages sometimes overtook me—I saw myself being pushed aside by another version of myself who was livid over something/nothing, and I would just stand back and watch. My poor, dear husband married an outspoken, independent, really nice girl. Just three years later, she turned into some sort of evil twin neither of us recognized. But she was living with us, so we had to deal with her.

I knew I had to understand what was happening and, as we do in Ayurveda, get to the root cause. I looked at my daily routine and examined every aspect. I was determined to be present for my menopause in a way that I was not during my raging puberty years. I wanted to pay attention, see what exactly was going on, and not shy away from the experience. It felt like something really important was happening to my body and mind, and I wanted to be there for it!

Through tears and fears I explained to my husband, Larry, that I was just exhausted and could not handle even the tiniest conflict, perceived conflict, or maybe just a word or a look. Or the sound of him chewing. Or snoring. All that threw me into a rage or sobs. I would feel the heat begin in my abdomen, like someone flicking on a furnace. It would spread in my chest and crawl up my face and scalp, enveloping me. This could happen as I drifted off to sleep, or began an engaging project, or in the car—the switch would flick, and my alter ego would arise like a phoenix from the flames.

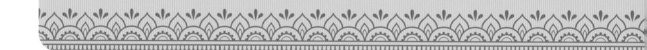

I finally understood that so much of this disturbance came from a lack of sleep: one or two hours, then boom, hot flash, covers off, window open. Then finally sleep again and boom, over and over and over again until I was in tears. Just a wreck. Sleep. I needed to sleep, then all would be better, I assured myself.

So how to get good sleep? I am an Ayurvedic practitioner! I should know this! But I was so busy helping others at the expense of my health. Finally, at this stage of life, I allowed myself to slow down for a minute, stop pushing forward so relentlessly, and heal myself.

Sleep is a culmination of everything that happens to you during the day. You need a balanced diet, movement, meditation, or some sort of mindfulness practice, and herbs and supplements if required. Ayurveda taught me to oil my body daily and massage my head and feet with cooling oil at night. I embraced all my practices, took the tools out of the toolbox, and used them. And to all this, I added a few drops of CBD/THC tincture before bed. Regretfully but productively, cutting out wine in the evening and coffee in the morning helped.

I came out the other side of menopause wiser, with more creativity and a drive for new adventures. I am so grateful for everything I went through, knowing that this stage of life is a passage into greater things. I began writing books post-menopause. I embraced new forms of creativity and expression. I opened up to my husband emotionally and sexually in ways I didn't even think were possible before. Menopause is just another doorway women pass through in life.

The reproductive system is never not important. Through every stage of life, we need to optimize nutrition and lifestyle to enhance and sustain the ability to assimilate nutrients into the deepest layers of our tissues. It's never too early to prepare for fertility, menopause, and andropause. The sooner we begin, the easier the transition will be.

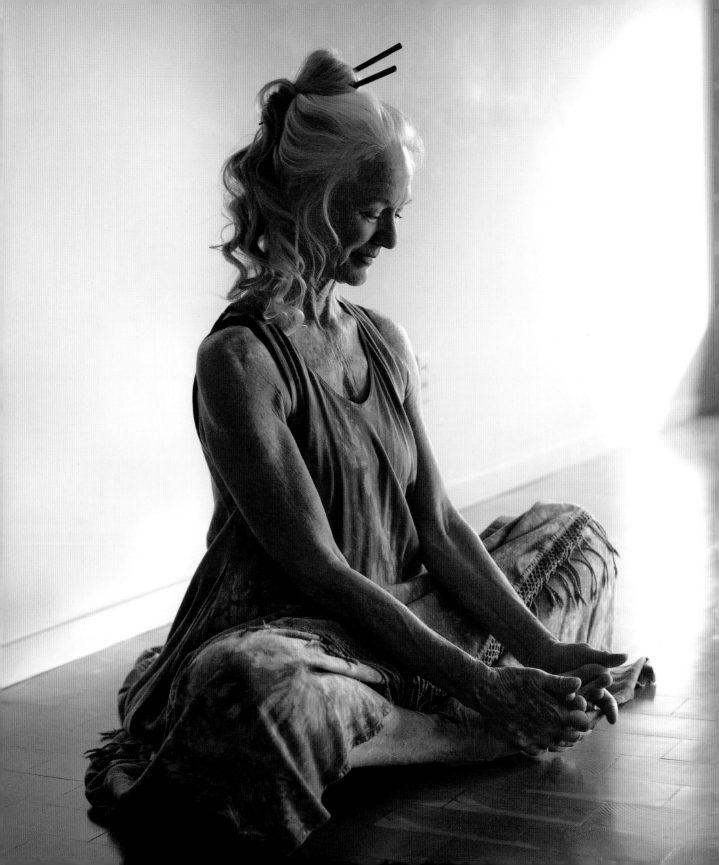

7

Caring for Yourself and Others at Every Age

Ayurveda offers remedies for issues that come up at every age, ideally building upon the practice, year by year, for every stage of life. The key is to maintain good diet, exercise, and lifestyle practices to reduce stress on the mind and body. Manage issues right away as they arise. Like Buddhism, Ayurveda suggests that the purpose of our practices is to die well—to be healthy until the end with our body and mind intact. I have witnessed death where the overtaxed body has given up. It simply shuts down, and the person is rendered unconscious with drugs meant to dull the pain and suffering. We don't want to die that way. We want to be present and aware as we take our final breaths. Dying well is a gift we give ourselves and our loved ones.

Aging Well

I've decided that I don't want to grow old gracefully. I want to grow old robustly! Graceful is not for me. I want to be swimming, dancing, walking, playing, lying in the grass—and able to get up without help. The key to this sort of longevity is elasticity. Be flexible, changeable, and adaptable in mind and body. If we get stuck in patterns or routines, such as believing limiting thoughts, staying in our lane, lacking imagination, eating the same foods season after season, we will get stuck. If we believe that aging means limits, contraction, and making our lives smaller, that is exactly what will happen.

I look at aging as expansion, openings, new beginnings, and adventures. Yes, we may have aches and pains in our joints from years of overuse—or from not enough use—accumulation of environmental toxins that we just could not avoid, and perhaps a limited income. There may be grief from loss and regrets. And loneliness as loved ones die. But with imagination and inventiveness, we may see the natural process of moving toward the end of life as a beautiful path.

FOOD: EATING FOR LONGEVITY

Choose food that supports your body. It is clear, and hundreds of studies show, that a diet high in sugar, bad fats, and processed foods contributes to diseases such as diabetes, cancer, obesity, and heart disease. They will shorten your life. A diet high in fresh fruits, fiber, vegetables, plant-based proteins, good carbs, healthy fat, fresh fish, and small amounts of meat will stave off disease and help you live longer.

LIFESTYLE: BREATH AS MEDICINE

Breathe to support your mind and body. All breath work is most effective on an empty stomach. Carve out 5 to 10 minutes a day for the practice of your choice, or use as needed. These techniques activate the parasympathetic nervous system, creating a wave of relaxation over the entire body.

There are contraindications to each technique, so please read thoroughly.

Vaidyagrama Morning Tea (aka Better Than Coffee!)

Many remedies in this book say to avoid coffee, but I know how hard that can be. Some of us may need to avoid coffee temporarily; for others, it may be forever. This tea is a morning ritual at the Vaidyagrama Ayurvedic center in India. The ginger and cardamom offer an intense flavor to wake you up, and the Indian sweetener jaggery (dried sugarcane) makes the tea feel like a treat. Before you drink, inhale deeply and smell the healing spices. This drink will fill your senses completely.

- 12–16 ounces (355–475 ml) fresh water
- 1 small green cardamom pod
- ½ teaspoon coriander seed
- ¼ teaspoon black pepper
- ¼ teaspoon ground ginger
- ½ teaspoon fennel seeds
- 1 teaspoon jaggery

Add all the ingredients, except the jaggery, to a pot and bring to a boil. Lower the heat and simmer for 5 to 10 minutes, depending on the strength you want; for a stronger tea, boil for longer. Pour into a mug through a fine-mesh strainer, then add the jaggery.

APOTHECARY: SUPPORTING AGING WITH ABHYANGA

Abhyanga massage. This is a wonderful everyday practice that feels especially luxurious in cold weather when our joints, bones, and tissues are craving the extra lubrication and warmth. Abhyanga penetrates the seven layers of our tissues—through the muscle, fat, nerves, blood, plasma, and bone—all the way to our reproductive organs, nourishing each layer along the way. The massaging action stimulates the lymphatic system, helping it pump toxins out of the body, as well as stimulating your own inner pharmacy and nourishing the skin's microbiome.

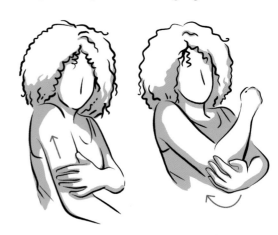

Ayurvedic massage oils blended specifically for each dosha are widely available online and in health food stores. Use only organic oils on the body. If you run cold, use the oils recommended for reducing Vata. If you run hot, use Pitta-reducing oil. If you feel thick and heavy, use Kapha reducing. Typically, we apply the oil before bathing, but after a bath or shower is fine, too.

Breath Work and Yoga Practice

SHEETALI/COOLING BREATH

To cool the mind and body, there is no better breath work than sheetali. This exercise brings cool air into the mouth, and heated air is expelled through the nose. Do this anytime it's needed. Count to ten to cool off; take ten sheetali breaths when aggravation, frustration, or impatience arises: Someone cuts you off in traffic; a workmate raises an old issue over and over again; your partner didn't do the dishes.

Teach your kids this technique (they love it because they can stick their tongue out!) to help them react with less intensity to "unfair" situations.

- Sit in a comfortable position with your chin level and eyes looking straight ahead, stick out your tongue, and roll it like a straw. (If you aren't able to curl your tongue read the next exercise). Inhale deeply through the curled tongue, pulling the cool air into your throat and down to your tummy. Follow the air as it cools the pathway deep into your body. After you have filled your belly with cool air, withdraw the tongue and place the tip of the tongue on the roof of the mouth behind the front teeth, close your mouth, and exhale through your nose. Notice how as the air exits the nose, it warms up, further helping you cool down. Repeat the process. Try six to ten rounds. If you feel dizzy, return to normal breathing.

SHEETKARI BREATH

This method is for those who aren't able to roll their tongues. With the same seated position, chin level, smile wide, and teeth slightly apart, place the tip of your tongue on the roof of your mouth just behind your front teeth, and pull air into your cheeks. Then close your mouth and exhale through the nose. Repeat six to ten times.

This cooling breath is contraindicated for those with constipation as it cools the nerves required for bowel contractions, exacerbating the problem. Do not try this if you have low blood pressure, asthma, or disorders of the heart. Practice only in the warmer months and avoid in cold climates.

ALTERNATE NOSTRIL BREATHING

Alternate nostril breathing has been called the ultimate breath work. Ayurveda says it heals just about anything from hot flashes and hormonal imbalances to depression, anxiety, and stress disorders. To practice, sit straight in a comfortable position. Place the tip of your tongue on the roof of your mouth, behind your front teeth.

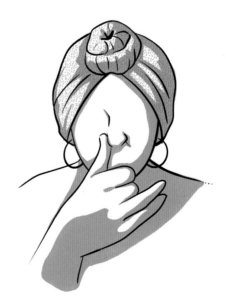

- Raise your right hand to your nose, keeping the pinky, ring finger, and thumb extended, and fold your index and middle fingers into the palm. Gently close your right nostril with your right thumb and inhale deeply through the left nostril, expanding your belly. Exhale fully through the same nostril keeping the right nostril closed, then inhale deeply again to the belly, and at the top of the inhale, close the left nostril with the right ring finger, open the thumb on the right, and exhale through the right nostril. At the end of the exhale, pause, then inhale deeply again through the right nostril, close your right nostril with your thumb and exhale left. Inhale left, close, and exhale right.

- To add extra benefit for grounding and stress reduction, pause between inhales, pinching both nostrils shut and holding your breath for 6 to 8 seconds, then release one side and exhale and continue the process.

- Try to do ten cycles. Each inhale/exhale is a cycle. If you feel dizzy, lower your hand and breathe normally. When you feel steady, begin again. Work your way up over time to twenty cycles.

Do not practice if you have a full stomach or high blood pressure.

BHASTRIKA

Bhastrika breath is the opposite of sheetali. It literally stokes the fires in the belly and the brain, helping to heat you up and wake you up! It's great for Kapha dosha and ideal to practice in winter or anytime you are feeling cold, dull, lethargic, and unmotivated. Known to increase lung capacity, Bhastrika dumps oxygen into the blood and facilitates the effective removal of carbon dioxide, which helps to cleanse and tone the tissues, blood, and cells. The intensity of the breathing clears the nasal passages and may eliminate constipation. Deep abdominal breathing increases and improves circulation.

- Sit comfortably with hands resting on your thighs or knees. Lower the shoulders to open your chest. Feel your spine elongate and sit straight but not rigid. Chin is level with the ground. Close your eyes and breathe normally through your nose. Have a tissue nearby as you may expel some mucus during the practice.

- Take several deep, full belly inhalations through the nose, exhaling through the nose completely. When you feel ready, take in a deep breath and forcefully expel the air on the exhale (all through the nose). Let the belly contract on the exhale, pushing the air out. Feel the belly button go back toward the spine. Your whole torso may even contract a bit. Then do a rapid, deep nasal inhale to the belly and forceful expulsion of air again.

- If this is your first time, do this for just three to five rounds to begin with and work your way up over days and weeks, getting up to ten cycles. No need to breathe rapidly as you begin the practice. Go slowly at first and work your way up to a faster practice. In the beginning, take one breath every 1 or 2 seconds. Don't push it. At the end of your practice, take a deep, slow inhale and a deep, slow exhale and relax, finding your natural breath. Sit quietly for a few minutes and feel how your body and mind have changed. You may feel tingles and feel more awake and aware.

If you don't have a teacher, try watching videos to master the technique.

This practice is quite intense and should not be done if you are pregnant or have your period. Do not practice this if you have glaucoma, high blood pressure, hernias, heart disease, or detached retinas or have had recent surgery, especially to the abdominal area. Bhastrika breathing is contraindicated for asthma, epilepsy, vertigo, or bronchitis or if you are at risk for stroke.

BOXED BREATHING

Boxed breathing is a gentle practice that calms you down, and helps you sleep or fall back to sleep. The process involves counting and visualizing, which increases concentration and helps you be fully in the moment.

- Be seated or lying down. Whichever your posture, begin with a few deep breaths through the nose to the belly. Let your tongue rise to the ridge behind the front teeth to relax your jaw and open your airways. Notice the gentle rise and fall of your chest or belly. Focus on bringing the inhale down to your belly and allowing it to expand like a balloon. When you feel ready, inhale to the count of four and visualize a straight line as you mentally begin to draw a box. At the top of the inhale, hold your breath for 4 seconds and draw the second line of your box. Exhale through the nose slowly to the count of four, and draw line three of the box. Holding your breath at the end of the exhale, pause for 4 seconds and complete the box drawing in your mind.

- Continue with the practice until you feel relaxed, focused, or sleepy, whichever outcome you are aiming for. Keep visualizing the box and keep the inhales and exhales steady and slow, through the nose, allowing for a gentle pause as you hold the breath between inhales and exhales.

There are no contraindications for this practice.

FORWARD BEND

This pose is deeply relaxing as well as rejuvenating. Encouraging the blood to flow to the brain, it's a great pose to refresh after work, bring enthusiasm and creativity to the forefront, or wash away a busy mind. This is a great pose for grounding and coming more deeply into yourself and the present moment.

- Stand with feet hip-distance apart and find your balance by focusing on the four corners of your feet: the pad under the big toe, the pad under the pinky toe, the right side of the heel, and the left side of the heel. If you need to, widen your stance. Place your hands on your hips, inhale through the nose, and exhale through the nose as you slowly bend forward from the waist, keeping the chin aligned with the floor as you move. As you deepen the bend, allow your head to gently fall forward, chin toward the chest, with the crown of your head toward the floor.

- Remove hands from the waist and gently clasp your elbows with the opposite hands. To deepen the pose, bring your palms to the floor or place your fingers under your toes. Knees should be soft. Bend slightly if that feels better. Sway a little, move your head and neck around, whatever feels comfortable with you. Stay in this pose as long as it's comfortable. Thirty seconds is a good amount of time.

To come up, bring your hands to your waist, keep your chin tucked, and slowly lift. The head should be the last to come up. Rise, one vertebra at a time. Breathe and allow your hands to fall to your side.

If you have blood pressure issues, hypertension, or glaucoma, avoid forward bends.

SUN SALUTATION

One of the best overall combinations of poses to exercise the entire body is the Sun Salutation. When done vigorously and repeated a dozen times or more, it is a true workout. But even four or five rounds will get your blood and breath moving. As the name signifies, this pose is perfect for welcoming the day. Face east and the rising sun energy will infuse the practice. Best done on an empty stomach or 2 hours after a meal.

- Place your feet slightly less than hip-distance apart, firmly on the ground. Head erect, ears over the shoulders, pelvis in neutral, bring hands up to your chest in prayer pose, thumbs against the heart chakra. Focus here and breathe in and out through your nose. On an inhale, reach for the sky, the upper arms close to the ears, palms facing each other. Slightly arch the back, moving the hips forward.

- On an exhale, lower your arms and bend forward, placing the hands alongside the outside of your feet. Bend your knees if you need to. Chin is toward the chest. Look out then look down again.

- Exhale and swing your right leg forward and plant the right foot under the right knee. Lower the left knee to the ground, toes on the left foot flexed. Look ahead and breathe.

- Push yourself up and swing the right leg back in line with the left leg, raise the hips, and come into downward dog. Your buttocks and hips move up into the air and your arms are outstretched in front of you at an angle. If possible, place your feet flat on the floor.

- Bring the hips down parallel to the floor, and on an exhale, swing the left leg forward, ankle aligned with the knee. Right knee comes to the ground for support. Hands flat on the floor next to the forward foot. Breathe.

- Inhale and swing the right leg next to the left and exhale and fold forward, palms on the floor into a forward bend. Bend knees if necessary.

- Inhale and bring the arms up, upper arms next to the ears, palms facing each other, slight arch in the back. Exhale and bring the hands down to the center of your chest in prayer pose. Rest, breathe, and repeat the sequence.

There are no contraindications for this practice.

SEATED YOGA STRETCHES

Perfect for times when we cannot stand for exercise, the movements here will give you all the benefits of Sun Salutations. These stretches are great in small places, like on an airplane, a train, or a park bench, in a hospital bed, or at home. It's a beautiful way to move the body and feel alive and well. We don't need to feel limited by our environment. Anytime we move, we begin to heal.

- Sit on a chair or the edge of a bed or couch. The spine is erect but not rigid. Feet are flat on the floor. If your feet don't reach the floor, place something sturdy beneath them, like a block, book, or pedestal.

- Bring your hands to prayer pose, thumbs against the heart chakra. Breathe in and out gently through the nose. Inhale and raise your arms up over your head and look up at your fingers. Feel the stretch in your neck and sides, extending the spine.

- Exhale and bring your hands down to your toes and lay your chest on your knees.

- Inhale and clasp your left knee, sit up straight, and bring it toward your chest, raising your chin and head to look up. Exhale and bring your nose toward your knee.

- Inhale and on the exhale, lower the leg and fall forward again, hands beside your feet. Keep hands down and look up, extending the spine. Lower the head, clasp the opposite knee, sit up, bring the knee to the chest, and look up. Exhale and bring your head down to your knee.

- Again, place the knee down, fold forward on an exhale, and put both hands next to your feet. Inhale and on the exhale, raise the arms up over the head, slightly arching the back. Hold here for two breaths, bring hands back to prayer pose, exhale, and rest. Repeat as often as it feels good.

  There are no contraindications for this practice.

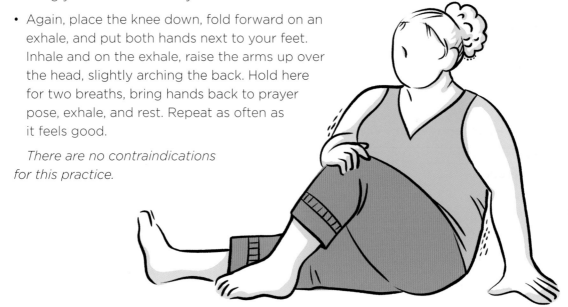

CHILD'S POSE

Children naturally fall forward and rest their heads and chests on the floor. Doing this pose as an adult brings those feelings of "floppy" back. Just resting. Being, not doing. Falling forward and into ourselves, this pose slows us down, gives permission to do nothing. Breathing slows naturally, and we rest. Do this pose anytime you feel unmoored, ungrounded, or overwhelmed. It's the perfect pose to do in between more challenging poses. As in all things in life, we need a period of rest to recover. Best to do on an empty stomach.

- Lower yourself to the floor to an all-fours pose, on hands and knees. Flex the spine in cat and cow a few times to loosen up. Inhale as you raise the hips up and round your back (cat), and exhale as you come down, belly toward the floor (cow). The head and chin come up on cow, and the chin tucks in cat.

- When you feel loose, bring your awareness to your breath, breathing in and out gently through the nose. Sit back and rest your buttocks on your heels.

- Spread your knees wide and allow your big toes to touch each other (if you are pregnant, only do this pose with knees spread wide, or avoid altogether). If it's uncomfortable to spread the knees, it's fine to keep them close.

- Sitting straight, extend the spine to its full length. Exhale and fall forward, bringing your torso toward the floor, between your thighs. Your forehead will come to the floor or to a block or blankets for support. Your chest will rest on your thighs.

- Extend your arms out, alongside your head, palms down, or keep them back and by your side, palms facing up. Keep your buttocks as close to your heels as possible. Place a rolled-up towel or blanket between your butt and your heels for support if needed.

- Rest, relax, and feel the stretch from the hips to the arms. Close your eyes. Breath normally.

- Feel the back open and expand with every breath. Stay in the pose as long as needed, or for at least 30 seconds.

- To release, walk your hands toward your torso, come upright to sit back on your heels.

- To get up from the floor, come back into tabletop by extending your arms and bringing the knees in. Walk your hands toward your feet and push up.

There are no contraindications for this practice.

Creating a Healthy Community

The system is not fair. People live in food deserts with no access to fresh, organic produce and affordable, healthy options. We know that sugar-laden fruit juice or sodas, processed foods, chemical preservatives, dyes, and excess salt make people sick. And when a pandemic hits, they are the first to suffer and die.

We are all in this together. If we do not address these issues, we are doing ourselves irreversible harm. So how do we find solutions and help each other?

- Ask for what you need by networking. Talk to your neighbors, friends, family, church, synagogue, or spiritual community. Social media sites such as Nextdoor and Facebook can be used to access goods and services that may not be readily available to you.

- Grow your own! Some herbs and leafy greens are able to be grown in your house on a windowsill or a balcony. Learn about vertical garden growing so you have your own fresh produce in your house.

- Join a community garden. Urban and suburban community gardens have established themselves around the country. If you don't have one near you, go online and learn how to start your own in your neighborhood.

- If you live in a food desert, try online shopping for what you need to be healthy. Learn where to order fresh produce and have it delivered to your door. For nonperishable items, try Vitacost, Eden Foods, and even Amazon. Order rice, beans, olive oil, coconut oil, natural soaps, shampoos, and more.

- Instead of buying wild-caught fish, which may be expensive, buy canned. Look for the safe-catch label.

- Organic produce is often pricey. Print out the lists of the Clean Fifteen and the Dirty Dozen from the Environmental Working Group (ewg.org). Use these guidelines to work within your budget and avoid pesticides.

- Local ethnic markets such as H Mart and Indian food stores have great prices and amazing food. Look for beans, spices, noodles, and rice that you may have never tried. A lot of the ingredients I write about in the remedies are in these stores.

Disease-Free Longevity for All

Ayurveda initially was known as healthcare for royalty, and it is still mainly accessible to the rich. I hope that this book will put power into the hands of all people. If you don't have time to do abhyanga massage every day, maybe find a couple of minutes to care for yourself. Start small and add what you can: A pinch of turmeric or ginger is well within reach. Drinking warm water with lime, instead of drinking soda, may be the start of subtle yet profound health benefits.

Please help me put this book and these ideas into the homes, hospitals, military bases, and schools for those who really need it. We are a team. Let's support each other along the way. Little acts will move us toward sustainable changes and healthy communities no matter where you live. This, my friends, increases longevity, boosts the immune system, and supports you in staying hearty and healthy as you age.

All the guidelines are here in the remedies for eating well, sleeping properly, eliminating toxins and waste, reducing stress and anxiety—fully healing your mind, body, and spirit. Rely on this book as a life manual and share it. Carry this timeless wisdom with you as you age robustly and help others along the way.

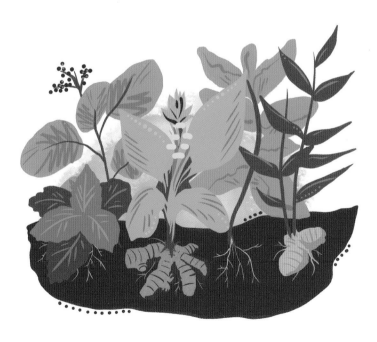

Resources

ARC underwear and more: Garments for all shapes and sizes, sewn in the US from certified organic, recycled, and/or deadstock materials. shoparq.com

Auromère toothpaste: auromere.com

Banyan Botanicals: banyanbotanicals.com

Blue Zones. How to live to 100: Recipes, lifestyle articles, secrets of longevity. bluezones.com

Coyuchi sheets and towels: Organic sheets, towels, and even nightwear. coyuchi.com

Dr. Bronner's organic body products: drbronner.com

Evanhealy skin care: Holistic, therapy-focused formulations. evanhealy.com

Himalaya products: himalayausa.com

Kerala Ayurveda: keralaayurveda.store

Maharishi Ayurveda: mapi.com

Organic India: organicindiausa.com

ProTren: Trustworthy probiotics. protren.com

Pukka Tea: pukkaherbs.com/us/en

Pure Indian Foods: pureindianfoods.com

Soapwalla: Handmade body products from the field to your body. soapwalla.com

CREATE YOUR OWN AYURVEDIC APOTHECARY KIT

Keep these herbs, spices, foods, and oils on hand so when a cough, cold, aches, or pains happen, you will have the remedies at the ready.

Aloe vera: gel for scrapes and minor burns, juice for regular bowel movements

Ashwagandha tablet or powder: stress relief, immune booster

Bhringaraj oil: for nightly application to head and feet to deepen sleep and relaxation

Boswellia tablet or powder: pain relief

Chyawanprash (Ayurvedic jam): immune booster

Coconut oil: daily oil pulling, antibacterial for mouth

Dosha-specific body oil: for daily/seasonal abhyanga massage

Dry brush: daily brushing to detox the lymph system

Ginger powder or root: digestive aid

Lavender essential oil: antifungal, antibacterial

Licorice powder: throat, cough, stomach, detox

Mahanarayan oil: aches and pains

Neem oil, tablet or powder: complexion, skin, detox, toothpaste

Raw, organic honey: sore throat, allergies, good gut health, skin scrapes, minor burns

Sesame seed oil: daily gargle, can be used for massage

Sitopaladi powder: cough and cold

Talisadi powder: cough and cold

Tea tree essential oil: antifungal, antibacterial

Tiger balm liniment: aches and pains

Tongue scraper: for removing bacteria from the tongue daily

Triphala tablets or powder: bowel movements, colon toner

Turmeric tablets or powder: anti-inflammatory

BOOK RECOMMENDATIONS

Breath: The New Science of a Lost Art by James Nestor

Clean: The New Science of Skin and the Beauty of Doing Less by James Hamblin

Prakriti: Your Ayurvedic Constitution by Robert Svoboda

The 3-Season Diet: Eat the Way Nature Intended by John Douillard

Body, Mind, and Sport: The Mind-Body Guide to Lifelong Health, Fitness, and Your Personal Best by John Douillard

The Ayurvedic Cookbook by Amadea Morningstar

The Ayurvedic Guide to Fertility: A Natural Approach to Getting Pregnant by Heather Grzych

Balance Your Hormones, Balance Your Life by Claudia Welch

The Everyday Ayurveda Cookbook: A Seasonal Guide to Eating and Living Well by Kate O'Donnell

This Is Your Brain on Food: An Indispensable Guide to the Surprising Foods That Fight Depression, Anxiety, PTSD, OCD, ADHD, and More by Uma Naidoo, MD

Acknowledgments

In 2008, Dr. Vasant Lad, the legendary founder of the Ayurvedic Institute, read my Vedic astrological chart. With wide eyes and a voice of wonder, he told me I was destined to become a major voice of Ayurveda in the West. Dr. Lad, we have spent so much time together in the past fourteen years, including six weeks in India. You gave me much courage and knowledge to be that voice.

Also in 2008, Amadea Morningstar called me an Ayurvedic poster child when I joined her for my first immersion into Ayurvedic cooking at the Kripalu Center for Yoga & Health in Stockbridge, Massachusetts, US. Amadea, you have been the greatest of mentors and kindest of friends.

Thank you to the hundred-plus people I have taken to India since 2007. You put your trust in my hands and welcomed India into your hearts. This could not have happened without Mr. Unni Nair and Mr. Sanjeev Joseph, of Royal Indian Voyages, my most trusted Indian friends and guides.

My friends and hosts at Vaidyagrama and Somatheeram, Ayurvedic centers in India: You have helped me introduce so many people to your ancient practices. Thank you for always attending to our health and taking such good care of us.

Marilyn Allen, my agent, is unfailingly supportive and positive of my ideas. I so appreciate all you do for me. And to my editors at Quarto Books/Fair Winds Press, Jill Alexander, Jenna Nelson Patton, Liz Weeks, and Maggie Cote. You took my words and thoughts and made them into something so comprehensive and beautiful! Such unwavering support you gave me as we navigated this together. I wish you could always be in my wake, fixing my words and making them pretty.

Larry, Ella, and Joonie, you provide for me the most loving home. We are surrounded by the healing powers of nature with the trees, birds, and all the forest creatures in our cozy space in the world. I could not do this without you.

About the Author

Susan Weis-Bohlen is an Ayurvedic consultant and writing teacher. She is the author of the best-selling *Ayurveda Beginner's Guide: Essential Ayurvedic Principles and Practices to Balance and Heal Naturally* and *Seasonal Self-Care Rituals: Eat, Breathe, Move, and Sleep Better—According to Your Dosha*. Susan began practicing, studying, and teaching Ayurveda after a profound personal experience with the Ayurvedic cleansing technique of Panchakarma. She has since studied with many of the top teachers of the practice including Deepak Chopra, Dr. Vasant Lad, and Amadea Morningstar. Susan has been on the board of the National Ayurvedic Medical Association (NAMA) since 2018. She regularly travels to India, introducing Ayurveda to hundreds of people over the years. Susan also leads destination Ayurveda and writing retreats around the world. She lives in Baltimore with her husband Larry and their dogs Ella and Joonie.

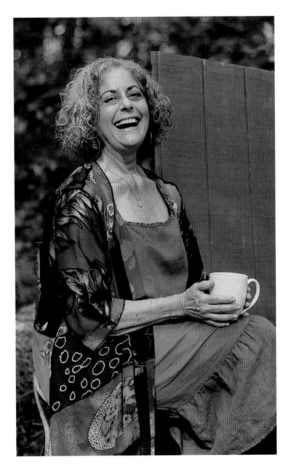

Index

A

aging
  abhyanga massage, 174
  alternate nostril breathing, 175–176
  andropause, 159–161
  ashwagandha, 150
  bhastrika breathing, 176–177
  boxed breathing, 177–178
  breathing, 172, 174–178
  child's pose, 181
  elasticity, 172
  foods and, 172
  forward bend pose, 178
  Kapha stage of life, 163
  menopause, 155, 162–169
  networking, 182
  pain, 46
  perimenopause, 162, 163
  Pitta stage of life, 163
  seated yoga stretches, 180
  sheetali breathing, 174–175
  sheetkari breathing, 175
  skin, 132
  Sun Salutation, 179
  Vata stage of life, 163

B

beverages. *See also* foods
  acid-reducing teas, 107
  alcohol, 30, 35, 37, 43, 91, 92, 98, 103, 106, 110, 111, 116, 126, 127, 133, 151, 153, 157, 160, 164
  Be Free of Allergies Smoothie, 84
  black tea, 35
  caffeine, 35, 83, 116, 127, 157, 164
  chamomile tea, 22, 28
  Cumin-Coriander-Fennel (CCF) tea, 37, 38, 41, 164

  dashamula tea, 55, 59
  dehydration, 51, 57, 71, 101–105, 133
  Extreme Hydration Smoothie, 104
  ginger tea, 50, 57, 71
  Golden Milk, 22, 24, 25
  gotu kola tea, 143
  green tea, 35, 71, 80, 85, 98, 119, 129, 151
  herbal tea, 24, 30, 35, 106, 111, 160
  hibiscus tea, 134
  Hot Flash Soother Smoothie, 165
  licorice tea, 37, 38, 71, 80, 134, 156
  manjistha tea, 134
  non-asthmatic breathing problems and, 71
  stinging nettle tea, 129
  talisadi tea, 74
  turmeric tea, 57, 71, 121
  Vaidyagrama Morning Tea, 173
  valerian root tea, 22, 28, 41
breathing. *See* respiratory system

C

conditions
  acid reflux, 105–110
  acne, 125–126, 144
  allergies, 81–85
  andropause, 159–161
  arthritis, 55
  bad breath, 94–95
  burns, 141–143
  Candida infections, 156–159
  colds, 70–75
  cough, 70–75
  dehydration, 101–105

  dry skin, 131–134
  gastric (peptic) ulcers, 118–121
  gastroesophageal reflux disease (GERD), 105–110
  headache, 51–54
  heartburn, 105–110
  high cholesterol, 96–99
  hives, 128–131
  hot flashes, 162–167
  infertility, 153–154
  insomnia, 30–36
  irritable bowel syndrome (IBS), 112–117
  joint pain, 55
  lower back pain, 56–59
  low libido, 150–153
  menopause, 162–169
  muscle aches and strains, 56
  neck pain, 54–55
  nightmares, 40–42
  non-asthmatic breathing problems, 70–75
  peptic ulcers, 118–121
  rashes, 128–131
  rhinitis, 76–81
  scars, 141–143
  seasonal conditions, 81–85
  sinusitis, 76
  sleep apnea, 37–39
  sore throat, 70–75
  sunburn, 127–128
  toenail fungus, 139–141
  vaginal dryness, 155–156
  vaginal yeast (*Candida*) infections, 156–159
  wounds, 141–143

D

digestion. *See also* foods
acid reflux, 105–110
agni, 87, 88, 94
ajwain, 74
ama, 156
Avipattikar churna, 109
bad breath, 94–95
bowel movements, 90, 113
clothing and, 108, 116, 121, 125
dehydration, 101–105
exercise and, 90
fennel seeds and, 121
gastric (peptic) ulcers, 118–121
gastroesophageal reflux disease (GERD), 105–110
ginger, 121
guggulu, 99
heartburn, 105–110
high cholesterol, 96–99
hing (asafoetida), 112
hormones and, 88
H. pylori, 118, 121
irritable bowel syndrome (IBS), 112–117
kanji, 120
licorice tea, 38, 106, 121
manda agni, 156
menopause and, 164
mental health and, 88, 91
microbiome, 89, 144
moringa, 121
oil pulling, 93, 95
oral microbiome, 92–93
peptic ulcers, 118–121
polyphenols, 119
psyllium husk, 99
shilajit, 99
sleep and, 91
slippery elm, 117, 121
stress and, 90, 108, 110
teeth, 92–93
triglycerides, 96
triphala, 91, 111, 117

turmeric tea, 121
vagus nerve, 88, 105, 117
visualization and, 108
weight loss, 111

F

foods. *See also* beverages; digestion; recipes
acid reflux and, 106
acne and, 125–126
aging and, 182
allergies and, 81–83
amalaki, 99
andropause and, 160
appetite, 22
bad breath, 94
blood flow and, 151
breakfast, 24
Breathe Free Soup, 72–73
burns and, 141
Candida infections and, 157–158
colds and, 70
cough and, 70
dehydration and, 102–103
dreaming and, 41
dry skin and, 132–133
ethnic markets, 182
fish, 21, 57, 67, 90, 97, 124, 148, 153, 160, 172, 182
food deserts, 182
gastric (peptic) ulcers and, 119
gastroesophageal reflux disease (GERD) and, 106
headaches and, 51, 52, 53–54
heartburn and, 106
high cholesterol and, 97–98
hing (asafoetida), 112
hives and, 129
hot flashes and, 164, 166
hydration and, 102, 125, 103, 132
infertility and, 153
insomnia and, 30
irritable bowel syndrome (IBS) and, 112, 116

junk foods, 124
kitchari, 114–115, 166
longevity and, 172
lower back pain and, 57
low libido and, 151
lunch, 24
menopause and, 164, 166
neck pain and, 54
nightmares and, 41
non-asthmatic breathing problems, 70
omega-3 fatty acids, 21, 67, 97, 124, 142
omega-6 fatty acids, 21
omega-9 fatty acids, 21
organic foods, 15, 39, 81, 90, 114, 159, 182
pain reduction with, 47
peptic ulcers and, 119
pesticides and, 182
prebiotics, 89, 90, 91, 103, 116, 119
probiotics, 89, 90, 91, 103, 116, 119, 145, 158
processed foods, 90, 111
pyramid, 48
rashes and, 129
reproductive system and, 151
respiratory system and, 67
rhinitis and, 80
root chakra and, 148
sacral chakra and, 148
saturated fats, 98
scars and, 141
seasonal conditions and, 81–83
skin and, 124, 127, 132–133, 142
sleep and, 21, 24, 30, 31, 35, 43
sleep apnea and, 37
snacking, 22, 43, 47, 98, 106, 110, 111, 119, 166
solar plexus chakra and, 148
sore throat and, 70
spicy foods, 129

sugar, 97, 98, 129, 139
sunburn and, 127
supper, 24
timing of, 24
toenail fungus and, 139
tryptophan in, 22
vaginal dryness and, 155
vaginal yeast (*Candida*)
    infections and, 157–158
weight loss and, 111
wounds and, 141
yogurt, 159

K

Kapha dosha
    abhyanga massage, 138
    appetite and, 22–23
    arthritis, 55
    bhastrika breathing, 176
    Candida infections, 156, 157, 158
    definition, 13
    dehydration and, 102
    digestive health, 22–23, 88, 112
    dosha quiz, 11–12
    dreaming, 40, 41
    elemental combinations as, 10
    ghee and, 164
    headaches, 53–54
    healing and, 13
    high cholesterol, 99
    hives, 130
    infertility, 154
    insomnia, 35–36
    introduction, 10
    irritable bowel syndrome (IBS),
       112
    joint pain, 55
    nightmares, 41
    oral care, 92
    pain response, 46
    personality, 13
    rashes, 130
    respiratory system, 66, 67
    rhinitis, 80
    skin care, 135, 137, 138

sleep, 30, 35–36, 37, 41, 42, 43
sleep apnea, 37
stage of life, 163
tongue and, 92
vaginal yeast (*Candida*)
    infections, 156, 157, 158
wash routine, 137
weight and, 101, 102, 111, 154

P

pain
    abhyanga massage, 50
    ajwain, 74
    awareness, 46
    body scan, 49
    causes, 46
    clothing and, 50, 58
    doshic response, 46
    exercise as response to, 49
    food for reduction to, 47
    headaches, 51–54
    hobbies as response to, 50
    joint pain arthritis, 55
    lower back pain, 56–59
    Marma therapy, 52, 53
    massage and, 50
    meditation and, 49, 60–63
    muscle aches and strains, 56
    natural relief, 50
    neck pain, 54–55
    Panchakarma protocol, 58
    professional advice, 49
Pitta dosha
    abhyanga massage, 138
    acid reflux, 105
    acne, 125
    andropause, 160
    appetite, 22–23
    arthritis, 55
    Candida infections, 156
    definition, 13
    digestive health, 22–23, 88, 91,
       105, 112, 118
    dosha quiz, 11–12
    dreaming, 40, 41

dry skin, 131
elemental combinations as, 10
gastric (peptic) ulcers, 118
gastroesophageal reflux
    disease (GERD), 105
ghee and, 164
headaches, 52–53
healing and, 13
heartburn, 105
infertility, 154
insomnia, 30–31
introduction, 10
irritable bowel syndrome (IBS),
    112
joint pain, 55
lunch and, 24
menopause, 163, 164
menstruation, 164
oral care, 92
pain response, 46
peptic ulcers, 118
personality, 13, 42
respiratory system, 66, 67
skin care, 131, 135, 136, 138
sleep and, 30–31, 40, 41, 42
stage of life, 163
tongue and, 92
vaginal yeast (*Candida*)
    infections, 156
wash routine, 136
weight and, 101, 154

R

recipes. *See also* foods
    Be Free of Allergies Smoothie,
       84
    Belly-Pacifying Kitchari, 114–115
    Breathe Free Soup, 72–73
    Cumin-Coriander-Fennel (CCF)
       tea, 38
    dashamula tea, 59
    Extreme Hydration Smoothie,
       104
    ginger tea, 50
    ginger-turmeric tea, 57

Golden Milk, 25

hibiscus paste, 134

hibiscus tea, 134

Hot Flash Soother Smoothie, 165

kanji, 120

kitchari, 114–115

licorice tea, 38, 71

Ojas Replenishing Treat, 152

Put Me to Bed Bathing
   Routine, 29

talisadi tea, 74

turmeric tea, 121

Vaidyagrama Morning Tea, 173

reproductive system

abhyanga massage, 154, 156, 167

alcohol and, 151

aloe vera juice and, 156

amalaki, 161

andropause, 159–161

aphrodisiacs, 150, 151, 153

ashwagandha, 150, 161, 167

Bhringaraj oil and, 167

blood flow and, 151

brahmi and, 153, 154, 167

Candida infections, 156–159

chamomile and, 167

clothing and, 149, 155, 158

gokshura, 153, 161

guduchi, 154

guggulu, 161

hot flashes, 162–167

infertility, 153–154

licorice and, 156, 161

love and, 150, 151

low libido, 150–153

menopause, 155, 162–169

ojas, restoration of, 152

perimenopause, 162, 163

root chakra and, 148

sacral chakra and, 148

safed musli, 151

shatavari, 149, 154, 156, 167

sleep and, 151, 154, 167, 169

solar plexus chakra and, 148

Triphala powder, 158

vaginal dryness, 155–156

vaginal yeast (Candida)
   infections, 156–159

valerian root and, 167

vetiver and, 167

vidari kanda, 154, 161, 167

weight and, 151, 154, 161

yogurt and, 159

respiratory system

aging and, 172

ajwain, 74

allergies, 81–85

alternate nostril breathing, 31,
   38, 41, 68, 119, 166, 175–176

antihistamines, 85

bad breath, 95

Be Free of Allergies Smoothie,
   84

bhastrika breathing, 36, 53,
   176–177

boxed breathing, 38, 41, 68,
   177–178

Breathe Free Soup, 72–73

Charaka Samhita on, 66

cleaning chemicals, 68

clothing and, 68, 69, 80, 83

colds, 70–75

cough, 70–75

deep breathing, 54, 66, 177

dosha ailment variations, 66, 67

environmental issues, 77, 80

essential oil steam, 75

gandusha (oil pulling) and, 69

hot flashes and, 166

insomnia and, 31, 36

kavala, 69

licorice tea, 71

longevity and, 172

masks, 69, 83

nasya oil for, 39, 82, 83

neti pot, 76, 78–79, 81, 83

non-asthmatic problems, 70–75

omega-3 fatty acids and, 67

quercetin, 69, 77, 85

rhinitis, 76–77, 80–81

seasonal conditions, 81–85

sesame seed oil for, 69

sheetali breathing, 30, 52, 68,
   95, 107, 119, 174–175

sheetkari, 175

sinusitis, 66, 76

sitopaladi powder, 71

sleep apnea, 37–39

sore throat, 70, 75

talisadi powder, 74

S

skin

abhyanga massage, 138

acne, 125–126, 144

alcohol and, 126

aloe vera, 134, 143, 145

antibiotics, 144

ashwagandha, 131

burns, 141–143

castor oil, 143

clothing and, 125, 127, 130, 142

dry skin, 131–134

Eladi Tailam blend, 130

exfoliating, 126

foods and, 124, 125–126,
   132–133, 139, 142

ghee, 143

gotu kola, 143

guggulu, 140

hibiscus, 134

hives, 128–131

injury care, 141, 143

licorice tea, 134

manjistha, 126, 134, 144

meditation and, 130

microbiome, 125, 142

neem, 126, 131, 133, 143, 145

oil pulling, 134

omega-3 fatty acids and, 124

over-washing, 125

rashes, 128–131

sandalwood, 128

scars, 141–143

sleep and, 133

stress and, 126
sunbathing, 125
sunblock, 128
sunburn, 127–128
supplements for, 134
tanning, 127
tea tree oil, 140, 143
toenail fungus, 139–141
triphala, 131, 140
turmeric, 126, 128, 140, 142, 143
vitamin C, 142
vitamin D, 127
washing, 125, 126, 131, 133,
    135–137, 140, 145
wounds, 141–143
zinc, 142
sleep
    abhyanga massage, 42
    acid reflux and, 107
    age and, 18, 19, 20
    aids for, 28
    alternate nostril breathing, 31
    bathing routine, 29
    benefits, 18, 20, 21, 43
    beverages and, 22, 24, 25, 28,
        37, 38, 41
    breathing and, 36, 38
    CBD/THC tincture, 169
    cholesterol and, 99
    circadian rhythms, 19
    clothing and, 42
    Cumin-Coriander-Fennel (CCF)
        tea, 38
    deep sleep, 18, 20
    didgeridoo and, 39
    digestion and, 91
    electronics and, 19, 27–28
    exercise and, 20, 36, 38
    fats and, 21, 24
    foods and, 21–22, 24, 30, 31, 35,
        37, 41, 43
    gastric (peptic) ulcers and, 121
    gastroesophageal reflux
        disease (GERD), 107
    Golden Milk, 25

    grounding and, 32
    head position, 27
    heartburn and, 107
    heart rate variability (HRV), 19
    insomnia, 18, 20, 30–33, 35–36
    journaling and, 27, 31
    libido and, 151
    light sleep, 18
    Marma therapy, 32, 33, 34
    massage, 34, 42
    melatonin, 19, 27, 28, 36
    memory and, 20
    menopause and, 167, 169
    monitoring, devices for, 19
    natural rhythm, 19
    nightmares, 40–42
    rapid eye movement (REM), 18
    reproductive system and, 151, 154
    sheetali breathing, 30
    skin and, 133
    sleep apnea, 37–39
    space for, 27, 42
    stages, 18
    support for, 19
    temperature and, 20, 27
    tryptophan, 22
    Vastu Shastra and, 27
    waking consciousness, 18

V

Vata dosha
    abhyanga massage, 138, 174
    andropause, 160, 161
    appetite and, 22–23
    arthritis, 55
    definition, 10
    digestive health, 22–23, 88,
        112, 118
    dosha quiz, 11–12
    dreaming, 40, 41
    dry skin and, 131, 133
    elemental combinations as, 10
    gastric (peptic) ulcers, 118
    ghee and, 164
    headaches, 51–52

    healing and, 13
    hot flashes, 163, 164, 167
    infertility, 154
    insomnia, 31–33
    introduction, 10
    irritable bowel syndrome (IBS),
        112
    joint pain, 55
    lower back pain, 56, 59
    menopause, 163, 164, 167
    oral care, 92
    pain response, 46, 50, 51–52,
        56, 59
    peptic ulcers, 118
    personality, 10
    Put Me to Bed Bathing
        Routine, 29
    respiratory system, 66, 67
    skin care, 131, 133, 135, 138
    sleep and, 30, 31–33, 40, 41, 42
    stage of life, 163
    tongue and, 92
    vaginal dryness, 155
    wash routine, 135
    weight and, 101, 154